the

VIBRANT LIFE

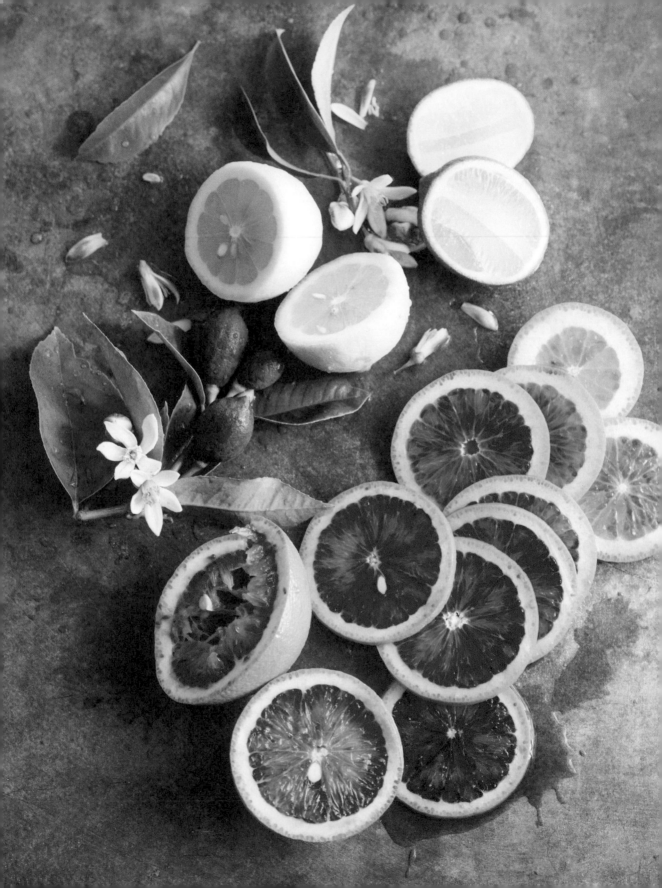

the

VIBRANT LIFE

EAT WELL, BE WELL

—

Recipes, Meditations, and Guidance on
Ways to Well-Being, from Acupuncture to Meditation

AMANDA HAAS

PHOTOGRAPHS BY ERIN KUNKEL

FOREWORD BY AYESHA CURRY

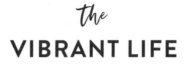

CHRONICLE BOOKS

SAN FRANCISCO

Library of Congress Cataloging-in-Publication Data:
Names: Haas, Amanda, author. | Kunkel, Erin, photographer.
Title: The vibrant life : eat well, be well /
Amanda Haas ; photographs by Erin Kunkel.
Description: San Francisco : Chronicle Books, [2019]
Identifiers: LCCN 2018033083 | ISBN 9781452170992 (hardcover : alk. paper)
Subjects: LCSH: Cooking. | Women--Nutrition. | LCGFT: Cookbooks.
Classification: LCC TX714 .H324 2019 | DDC 641.5--dc23
LC record available at https://lccn.loc.gov/2018033083

Manufactured in China.

FSC
www.fsc.org

MIX
Paper from
responsible sources
FSC™ C008047

Design by Sara Schneider.
Food styling by George Dolese and Elisabet der Nederlanden.
Prop styling by Glenn Jenkins.

Chronicle books and gifts are available at special quantity discounts to corporations, professional associations, literacy programs, and other organizations. For details and discount information, please contact our premiums department at corporatesales@chroniclebooks.com or at 1-800-759-0190.

10 9 8 7 6 5 4 3 2 1

Chronicle Books LLC
680 Second Street
San Francisco, California 94107
www.chroniclebooks.com

To Connor and Charlie, the constant loves of my life. Every day I wake up, I hope I show you what it means to be connected to your passion in life. I love you, my sons.

CONTENTS

FOREWORD 8

CREATING A VIBRANT LIFE

My Story 10

My Food Philosophy 14

My Feel-Good Ingredients 16

My Must-Have Tools 17

Chapter 1:
My Best Breakfasts, Hot Drinks, and Juices   21

Maple-Turmeric Golden Milk 22

Coconut-Almond Matcha 23

Chai-Spiced Cashew Milk 24

"Haascai" Berry Shakes or Bowls....................25

Meyer Lemon and Asian Pear Juice with Mint 26

Sophia's Toasted Almond Granola with Cardamom and Chocolate Chunks 27

Strawberry-Basil Smoothies with Almond Milk and Honey 29

Sheet-Pan Smoky Sweet Potato Hash with Oven-Roasted Eggs 31

Almond Flour Banana Bread with Dark Chocolate Chunks 33

Crustless Mini-Quiches with Roasted Red Pepper, Basil, and Goat Cheese 35

Buckwheat Crêpes with Berry Compote and Maple-Whipped Goat Cheese 36

"Stir-Fried" Quinoa and Greens with Poached Eggs, Avocado, and Salsa Verde.................38

On Mind Body Spirit   40

The Healing Properties of Yoga with Lindsey Valdez 41

Ingredients for Longevity with Rebecca Katz, MS.................................52

Time in Nature... 61

Massage Therapy for Self-Care 63

Talk Therapy 68

Chapter 2: Vegetables, Fruits, and Other Delicious Plants   71

Strawberry-Arugula Salad with Toasted Almonds and Mint..72

Napa Cabbage Salad with Fennel and Roasted Almonds 73

Butter Lettuce Salad with Asian Pears, Pistachios, and Pomegranate Seeds 75

Modern Salade Niçoise with Poached Tuna and Curry Aioli Dressing.................................77

Warm Spinach Salad with Beets, Apples, and Bacon Vinaigrette 79

Late Summer Salad with Heirloom Tomatoes, Stone Fruit, Goat Cheese, and Pistachios 81

Green Bean and Snap Pea Salad with Mustard Vinaigrette.................................83

Thai Rice Noodles with Peppers and Asparagus 85

Seamus's Butternut Squash Soup with Garlicky Panko Crumbs 88

Lentil Minestrone with Chard, White Beans, and (Sometimes) Sausage 90

Blistered Curry Cauliflower with Mint, Currants, and Toasted Almonds 93

Cauliflower-Kale Soup with Toasted Pine Nuts..........95

Merritt's Sexy Cannellini Beans (a.k.a. Almost-Vegetarian Cassoulet)................................97

Shaved Brussels Sprouts with Root Vegetables and Citrus–Goat Cheese Vinaigrette 99

Fall Quinoa Salad with Butternut Squash, Toasted Pepitas, and Raisins.................................101

Zucchini "Spaghetti" with Corn and Cherry Tomatoes....................................103

Wild Rice Salad with Butternut Squash, Cherries, and Mint..105

On Mind Body Spirit   106

The Medicine of Humor with Dr. Jennifer Aaker and Naomi Bagdonas 107

Strength Training for Total Body Fitness with Denise Henry 111

Cryotherapy 120

Sex and Aging with Pepper Schwartz 122

The Benefits of Acupuncture........................128

Chapter 3: Land and Sea — 131

Chicken in Lettuce Cups with Crispy Pine Nuts and Lime..........133

Chicken Pho with Daikon "Noodles" 137

Roasted Moroccan Chicken with Cauliflower "Couscous"..........139

Sticky Orange Chicken with Caramelized Onions and Fennel..........142

Thai Chicken Burger with Pickled Papaya Slaw..........144

Pork and Mango Stir-Fry with Napa Cabbage and Toasted Almonds 146

Sweet Potato–Turkey Chili with Cilantro Oil and Pepitas..........149

Pork Chops with Mashed Sweet Potatoes and Cranberry Sauce 151

Grilled Rib Eyes with Hasselback Sweet Potatoes and Preserved Lemon Gremolata 155

Steak Tacos with Cabbage Slaw, Mango Salsa, and Chipotle Mayonnaise 157

Coconut Ginger Sea Bass in Parchment with King Trumpet Mushrooms and Bok Choy..........160

Tuna Poke with Miso Mayonnaise and Pickled Cucumber..........163

Ceviche with Grilled Pineapple, Tomatillos, and Jalapeño..........167

Pan-Seared Scallops with Citrusy Corn Succotash 168

Whole-Roasted Fish with Currant Brown Butter Sauce..........170

Coconut Thai Prawns with Turmeric and Ginger..........172

Chapter 4: Sweets, Treats, and Cocktails — 175

Gluten-Free Ginger Molasses Cookies 177

Stone Fruit and Berry Crisp..........178

Greek Frozen Yogurt with Luxardo Cherries and Dark Chocolate Chunks..........179

Chocolate Ganache Tart with Grand Marnier 181

Matcha Panna Cotta 183

Summer Berry Pot Pies..........187

Orange-Tarragon Granita 190

Tequila Old-Fashioneds with Luxardo Cherries..........191

Herb Garden Gin and Tonic 192

Sauvignon Blanc Sangria..........194

Amanda's California Cocktail..........195

On Mind Body Spirit — 196

The Power of Group Exercise with Stephanie Peters and Sumner Weldon..........197

Love the Skin You're In with Kelly Hood 201

Meditation for Self-Love with Hailey Lott..........207

Sleep for Your Health..........215

Chapter 5: Twelve Staple Recipes That Get Me Through the Week — 219

Salsa Verde..........220

Preserved Lemon Gremolata..........221

Herb Buttermilk Dressing 222

Lemon Vinaigrette 223

Lime Vinaigrette..........224

Curry Aioli Dressing 225

Cucumber Salad with Mint, Red Onion, and Chinese Five Spice..........226

Mustard Vinaigrette..........228

Tamari, Ginger, and Honey Marinade (a.k.a. Amanda's Weeknight Marinade)..........229

Perfect Chicken Stock 230

Basic Quinoa..........231

The Perfect Poached Egg..........232

ACKNOWLEDGMENTS — 233

REFERENCES — 234

INDEX — 236

FOREWORD

Amanda Haas is the first person who encouraged me to put my recipes in writing and start creating a cookbook. At the time, I was shy about it. I knew I could cook, but it's one thing to cook at home for the ones you love and quite another to share your work with the world for critique. (It's nerve-racking, to say the least!)

One day, at Amanda's request, I shared some of my writing and recipes with her. Immediately, she got me. The thing that sealed our friendship? She understood that I had something to give the food community that was completely my own—my own recipes, my own stories, and my own combinations of ingredients. What Amanda told me that day has held true: the culinary world would make room for me because I had my own unique point of view on cooking and could articulate it. She is always saying, "There is room for everyone!" And she was right. The culinary world opened its arms wide for me and welcomed me into the fold.

As our culinary careers have taken off, Amanda and I have been lucky enough to anchor each other. Even in our busiest times, we've found ways to connect over food. Even though our lives look a little different on the outside—Amanda would tell you she's not married to an NBA player and she's definitely past having more children!—we share so much in common: We are both getting food on the table for our families; we run a million miles an hour; and we say yes to work that takes us in dozens of directions at once. We also simply love to cook. Whenever we come together through our work—whether it's prepping Christmas dinner together and then serving it separately for our family gatherings or creating a special cocktail together for a demo—we share our experiences, learn from each other, and get to see where this crazy world of food has taken each of us.

Amanda's mission in the food world has remained consistent. She wants to improve the way we eat and help people understand the connection between what we eat and how we feel. It's personal for her, as she has learned over the years that some foods make her feel incredible, but other foods can literally make her sick. She has spent the last decade learning about the American diet, what consuming so many refined and processed ingredients is doing to us, and how we can reverse some of the negative health effects of what we eat.

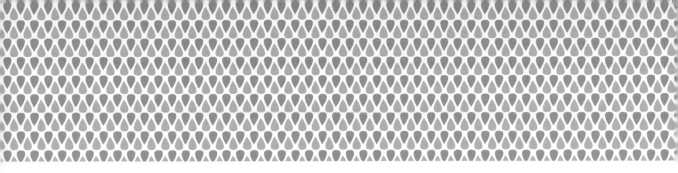

What I love about Amanda's approach to food and wellness is that she has done the homework for us. Through all her research, she holds the firm belief that food—even food that is ridiculously good for us—should taste good! Nothing else matters if it's not delicious.

Her last book, *The Anti-Inflammation Cookbook*, garnered well-deserved attention because it brought an important problem to light—that chronic fatigue, pain, and other disabling symptoms can be the result of exposure to foods that cause inflammation—and provided a solution through tasty, thoughtful recipes and accessible information. This time, Amanda has gone even further by looking outside of the food world to see what else we need to live our best lives and feel great.

If there is one thing to say about Amanda, it's that she's passionate about her quest to feel great and live a balanced life—and to help others do the same. (She is constantly trying to drag me to her favorite cycling class or hole-in-the-wall establishment for acupressure foot massages!) I knew the food in this book would be good—hellooo Matcha Panna Cotta!—but beyond that, I am so grateful to have a book that helps me understand what's going on with my body as I age, and what it needs to thrive. This is my new resource for pursuing all different elements for well-being, and I can't wait to share it with all the important women in my life.

Thank you, Amanda, for creating a book that will be treasured forever!

—Ayesha Curry

CREATING A VIBRANT LIFE

MY STORY (OR, WHY AM I WRITING THIS BOOK?)

Every morning, I wake up and begin my ritual. I press "snooze" and sink back into my bed, murmuring, "I love it here." I'm referring to my bed and my house, as they're both fairly new to me. After talking myself out of a second snooze, I pull myself out of bed and conduct that self-critique in the mirror that most women are capable of in less than one second. The question I ask myself is:

"How do I look today?"

It's a superficial question for sure, and each day I'm comparing myself to the last. For the most part, I'm happy with what I see. Today, my abs look pretty flat, my legs look strong, and my wrinkles are at an acceptable level. My eyes are clear, and I like what I see when I look in them. I see honesty, and a little lingering sadness after a period of extreme change in my personal life, but I am happy to wake up and start my day and it shows. I mentally rate myself a solid "8.0" before moving on to my next task.

By the time I walk to the bathroom and look in the mirror again, my mind automatically moves to question number two:

"How do I *feel* today?"

Until recently, the truthful answer was I felt lousy. I ached everywhere—I'd become accustomed to relentless, gnawing pain after thirty years with back injuries—and my joints were hurting constantly. My newly acquired muffin top was not lost on me, and my face and fingers were puffy. Then I remembered I woke up really hot in the middle of the night. And as I continued on with my day, a familiar feeling of anxiety set in, the type that fuels me to run around all day, but then feel like I've accomplished nothing. (Think laundry, getting my boys to clean their room, attempting a workout, a few minutes of meditation, a busy workday, and three hours spent commuting.) It left me short-tempered and slightly annoyed as the day wore on.

Frankly, I was spinning like a top, and my body was trying to tell me so. When my head hit the pillow, I'd be out cold one minute, then awake the next. Or I'd wake up thinking it's the morning and discover it's only 2:00 a.m., then lie awake for a few hours before falling back to sleep. It was a continual cycle of chronic fatigue. And as I sat down to write this book, I realized I've been asking myself the wrong questions. At forty-five, I'd had plenty of time to settle into my body, and somewhere deep in my mind, I realized I had probably reached the halfway point in my life. So I stopped, finally, and thought about the question I *should* be asking myself:

"What do I *want* out of this body?"

I'm not looking to turn back the clock. Aside from the aches and pains I experience, I love that age has provided me with a stronger sense of self, courage, and compassion. But what I want is to feel great. Not simply to be alive and going through the motions, but to feel *great*. I want energy, a positive outlook, motivation to be my best self every day, and a body that reflects it. I want great love in my life, in all forms and from all kinds of people. When I meet someone new, I want them to think, "Amanda is the absolute best version of herself."

But at forty-five, should I assume I've already peaked physically? Do people really have to feel worse as they age? Can't I start to feel better as I age, or at least slow down the clock a little? As I started to write this book, a few people showed up in my life to challenge my beliefs about aging.

There was Jackie, an eighty-year-old divorced mother of six. I met her on a flight from New York to San Francisco. When Jackie isn't trotting the globe or painting her second home herself, she's teaching yoga, meditating, participating in her political discussion club, and tooting around San Francisco in a powder-blue Mini Cooper. She shared a story with me about her eightieth birthday, where she hired a yoga instructor to lead a class for four generations of her family. Clearly, Jackie has decided that her health can flourish as she ages.

There was Seamus Mullen, a well-known New York chef who was diagnosed with rheumatoid arthritis. In 2013, he was so symptomatic he wound up in the hospital with a fever of 106°F [41°C]! After surviving that ordeal, Seamus made the decision to reject his life sentence of disease and helplessness. At forty-four, he is unrecognizable next to a photo of him from his early years of the disease. He's lost fifty pounds, is an avid yoga enthusiast, works out daily,

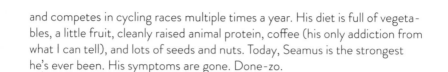

and competes in cycling races multiple times a year. His diet is full of vegeta-bles, a little fruit, cleanly raised animal protein, coffee (his only addiction from what I can tell), and lots of seeds and nuts. Today, Seamus is the strongest he's ever been. His symptoms are gone. Done-zo.

Then there was Dr. Pepper Schwartz. Within the first twenty-four hours of meeting this vibrant seventy-two-year-old professor and television person-ality, I attended her lecture on sex to a group of fifty, and was later doing a Zumba class next to her when she asked me, "How many of these people do you think actually know how to use their hips?" (You get the picture. This woman is having FUN.) As a tenured professor at the University of Wash-ington, relationship expert on the hit show *Married at First Sight*, and the author of twenty-five books on the subjects of love and sexuality, Pepper is the coolest, most lively, and most accomplished woman I know. She lives on a horse ranch that she built, and she rides daily when she's home. She travels for adventure and balances a rich personal life with teaching and lecturing all over the world. Pepper's life at seventy-two is what I want my life to look like right now!

After meeting these three phenomenal humans, I was forced to look at their similarities. They aren't defined by their age, and they've chucked standard beliefs about aging and health out the window. They've all discovered that they can actually feel *better* as they age.

Inspired, I dove into the world of living well. I've always known that cooking can improve how I feel, but I opened myself up to areas that I had neglected or simply didn't know about before. From acupuncture to meditation to cryotherapy—yes, I tried it!—I have spent the past year exploring all types of practices to feel my absolute best.

In the process, I discovered I had a tumor on my parathyroid gland that was causing me a lot of pain and health troubles. I needed surgery to remove it. (Go to the doctor regularly and get bloodwork done.) I also was having extreme reactions to foods, causing joint pain, redness, and welts all over my chest and head. My lower-back injury reared its head and I could not walk for two weeks. This led to—you guessed it—another surgery the same year! As I healed, I decided to dig into the habits I'd heard could improve my health, but had never been able to commit to consistently. Yoga, meditation, and walking

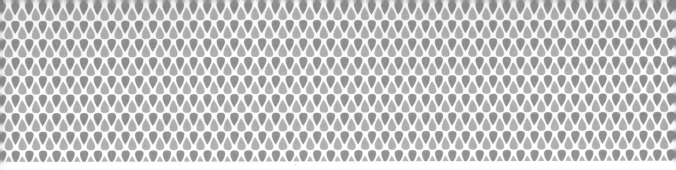

all became regular habits in my day. I started taking a cycling class consistently. I thought seriously about my wine intake and decided to stop drinking for a while. Lo and behold, I started to feel alive and vibrant again.

The results have been dramatic. Following the recipes and practices found in this book, I lost fifteen pounds, the payoff of making the time to push myself to eat better and stop making excuses for not moving more. I'm cultivating happy, healthy relationships and letting go of the ones that were keeping me from being my best self. My energy is back. I'm strong for once! I laugh all the time. I have perspective. Now, like Jackie, I can look in the mirror and say I feel as good as I did twenty years ago. And I probably look it, too, because I feel great in my skin. My body no longer reflects how I thought I'd feel at this age; it feels so much better than I could have imagined.

I hope you'll take one thing away from this book: we are all unique and need different things to feel great. As Dr. Pepper says, "We are not all the same age at the same age." It's up to you to figure out the formula for your own well-being, and to fully embrace it whatever your age! Whether it's meditation, yoga, cooking (always for me!), sleep, therapy, group exercise, nature, laughter, or a combination of many things, I hope this book gives you the tools you need to live your best life.

The real person I dedicate this book to is you.

With love,

Amanda

MY FOOD PHILOSOPHY

I live and eat in the real world, so everything in this book is how I strive to eat daily.

Because I have had food sensitivities and allergies my whole life, there are certain foods I will never touch again, like those that include gluten. But like most people, I allow myself to have almost everything in moderation so that I don't feel deprived. (There are plenty of nights that you'll find me enjoying really good ice cream or a glass of red wine.) The recipes you'll find in this book are how I want to cook at home, as they're full of flavor without a ton of refined, junky ingredients.

An anti-inflammatory diet is also an ageless diet.

In 2016, I decided to tackle anti-inflammatory cooking because I'd spent years with stomach pain, heartburn, and back and neck problems. As I improved my diet, I physically started to feel so much better that anti-inflammatory cooking became the foundation for my eating habits today. The anti-inflammatory ingredients I use will be the pillars in this book as well, as my anti-inflammatory diet has been the key to helping me feel great daily. The better I eat, the better I feel. Eating right not only makes me feel better inside, but also age better. I hurt less, I have more energy than I've had in a decade, and my skin looks better than it has in years. In case you didn't read my last book—no hurt feelings—let me catch you up on inflammation:

Inflammation is the body's response to outside irritants and stresses. It's a natural part of our immune system, and without it our wounds wouldn't heal. But when chronic inflammation occurs, it upsets our internal ecosystems, wreaking havoc on our digestive and nervous systems. Innumerable factors bring on chronic inflammation, and more and more people are becoming aware of its effects, electing to eliminate known irritants, such as gluten, in an effort to feel better. Yet while gluten sensitivity has gone mainstream, gluten is not the only irritant causing chronic inflammation. The typical Western diet of processed foods, excessive sugar, regular alcohol consumption, and too little of the foods that naturally counter inflammation, such as fresh vegetables, seeds, nuts, and oily fish, is contributing greatly to widespread chronic inflammation.

Chronic inflammation can prompt or worsen heart disease, inflammatory diseases (i.e., rheumatoid arthritis, lupus, celiac disease), diabetes, and many diseases (the list is long). In its lesser form, chronic inflammation can manifest as gastrointestinal upset, lethargy, or overall malaise. (I had all of these symptoms when consuming gluten and dairy and sugar to a lesser extent.) You'll see cancer frequently referenced in the information about beneficial and problematic foods. Put very simply, cancer loves inflammation, so reducing systemic levels of inflammation can be one way to positively manage or possibly prevent cancer. As a first step, informed, intentional eating can play a material role in promoting overall wellness and curbing the onset or progression of diseases that are negatively affected by inflammation.

I eat the foods that work best for my body.

I feel best when eating tons of green foods, lots of lean animal proteins, very little dairy, and zero—I mean zero—gluten, so that's what you'll find in this book. Even if you feel fine with gluten, dairy, and other "hot topic" ingredients, I encourage you to try life without them for a few weeks and listen to your body. Sweeteners are another charged food issue; natural or minimally refined sweeteners—honey, maple syrup, date, coconut, and natural cane sugars—are my go-tos.

I eat as organically as possible.

Yes, it costs more, but the difference in how you feel can be life-altering. Try to eat as much organic food as possible, and eliminate the so-called Dirty Dozen first. These are the twelve fruits and veggies that absorb the most pesticides during the production cycle, listed here in order from worst offender to least worrisome:

· Apples	· Peaches	· Cucumbers
· Strawberries	· Spinach	· Cherry tomatoes
· Grapes	· Sweet bell peppers	· Snap peas (imported)
· Celery	· Nectarines	· Potatoes

I limit refined foods, artificial anything, and alcohol.

This is common sense prevailing. I have yet to meet a doctor or leader in the food world who argues that refined foods make you feel good or age well.

Simply put, I want to make food taste so good, you don't ask what's missing!

MY FEEL-GOOD INGREDIENTS

PERISHABLES

- Alliums: garlic; green, red, and yellow onions; shallots
- Almond milk or cashew milk (homemade whenever possible)
- Avocados
- Beef (grass fed and organic)
- Brassicas: broccoli, Brussels sprouts, cabbage, cauliflower, Romanesco
- Butter (grass fed, such as Kerrygold)
- Carrots
- Celery
- Chicken (free range and organic)
- Citrus fruits: lemons, limes, oranges, and tangerines
- Eggs (free range and organic)
- Fish
- Fresh herbs: parsley, mint, chives, basil, thyme
- Kefir
- Lettuces and greens: kale, arugula, and chicories

PANTRY STAPLES

- Canned beans: black beans, chickpeas, pinto beans
- Chicken stock (homemade whenever possible)
- Coconut aminos
- Coconut milk
- Coconut oil
- Coffee
- Dijon mustard
- Gluten-free flours: almond flour, brown rice flour, natural blends (such as Bob's Red Mill)
- Olive oil
- Quinoa
- Spices: cinnamon, cloves, curry powder, fennel seeds and powder, ginger, nutmeg, oregano, red pepper flakes, turmeric
- Spirits: red wine, tequila, vodka (all used in limited amounts)
- Sweeteners: honey, maple syrup, raw natural cane sugar
- Tamari
- Vinegars: balsamic, red wine, sherry, white wine

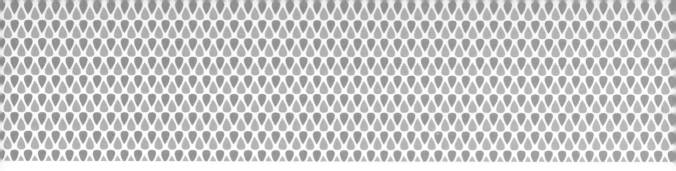

WHAT YOU WON'T FIND HERE

- Products containing gluten
- Cow's milk (I use milk and cream very sparingly when baking or making my kids' favorite pasta. I do much better with goat's milk.)
- Packaged products with long ingredient lists
- Products with food coloring

MY MUST-HAVE TOOLS

No matter what type of cooking I'm doing, I go back to the same tools time and time again. You don't need many! I bought most of these tools when I started working with Williams-Sonoma more than twenty years ago. I love looking in my drawer and finding many of the originals still there. If you're looking to build a kitchen with the most necessary tools, or update your collection, here's my list.

- **Blender:** Look for a high-speed blender with a very powerful motor, such as a Vitamix or KitchenAid. (I think it's worth the investment.)

- **Citrus press:** I have a handheld press that fits lemons and limes. It comes in so handy when making vinaigrettes and sauces, and adding citrus directly to a pan sauce.

- **Colander:** I have had a 12 in [30.5 cm] stainless steel colander for twenty years and it's perfect for draining pasta, rinsing beans, or scrubbing the dirt off of vegetables.

- **Cookware:** When it comes to cookware, I say invest early and reap the benefits of high quality. I still have the All-Clad I bought over twenty years ago and it works perfectly. I love my Hestan NanoBond cookware. My favorite pans to have: a 6 to 8 qt [5.7 to 7.5 L] Dutch oven, a 3 qt [2.8 L] stainless-lined sauté pan, a 10 in [25 cm] nonstick skillet, a 4 qt [3.8 L] saucier or braiser, a 3 qt [2.8 L] saucepan, and an 8 to 10 qt. [7.5 to 9.5 L] stockpot.

- **Cutting board:** Make sure you have a few. I have one that is thin and easily washable for fish and meat prep, and a thick, wooden one that is big enough to prep a ton of ingredients at once.

- **Dry measuring cups and spoons:** My friend Phil Rose designed what I consider to be the most amazing dry measuring cups and spoons of all time for Williams-Sonoma. The measuring spoons nest inside the cups, so they take up very little space in my drawer. Game changer.

- **Fine-mesh sieve:** I use a sieve to remove the layer of foam from stocks, or to remove anything that is so fine a colander wouldn't catch it.

- **Fish spatula:** It is so poorly named because a "fish spat" is capable of so much more than just flipping fish. I use my thin, flexible spatula to flip just about anything from flaky fish to veggies to pancakes.

- **Food processor:** I am in love with my Breville food processor. It has adjustable blades to slice tomatoes as thin as paper, shredding blades for veggies and cheese, a dough blade for breads and pizza doughs, and a few other incredible attachments. No matter what brand you select, you want a food processor that is heavy with a nice assortment of blades.

- **Knives:** As with my cookware, I believe in buying the best knives and taking great care of them. I regularly use a sharpening steel, and have them professionally sharpened when necessary. My basic assortment consists of a 6 in [15 cm] santoku, an 8 in [20 cm] chef's knife, a serrated knife for bread and thin-skinned fruits, and a 3½ in [9 cm] paring knife.

- **Liquid measuring cups:** OXO makes liquid measuring cups that show the volume of the liquid up the sides of the cup inside the cup, so you can see how much you're actually pouring as you work. Brilliant.

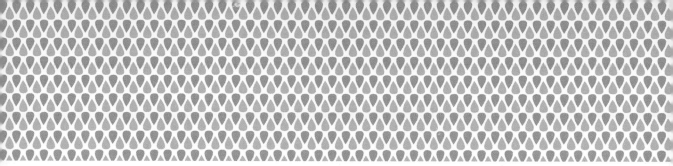

- **Microplane or zester:** I use my Microplane zester for all types of tasks. It grates things so finely that they practically melt into your food. Use it to zest citrus fruits, to finely grate Parmesan cheese, chocolate, or ginger, and to make garlic so fine that the pieces dissolve into your sauce. (Whenever a recipe calls for mincing garlic, I prefer to grate it.)

- **Mixing bowls:** I prefer metal bowls with wide, flat bottoms for stability.

- **Sheet pans:** I use USA Goldtouch sheet pans to roast just about everything, including all of the vegetables you'll find in this book. I like two sizes: the "half sheet" (13 by 18 in [33 by 46 cm]) and the "quarter sheet" (9 by 13 in [23 by 33 cm]) sizes. You can purchase great nonstick ones if you like, or stick with aluminum and line them with parchment paper for baking.

- **Spoons and spatulas:** I use metal, wood, and silicone spoons and spatulas when I'm cooking. If I'm cooking something over a very high heat, I stick to wood. If I'm using a nonstick pan, I still lean toward wood or silicone even though most nonstick is now scratch resistant. I prefer metal for big batches of chili, stock, or braises.

- **Tongs:** These need to be sturdy and easy to open and close. For me, the simpler the design, the better. I love the OXO tongs because they lock on the end for easy storage, and they have stay-cool edges on the handles so you don't burn yourself when holding them around an open flame. Brilliant!

- **Whisk:** You only need one or two. I like a bigger balloon whisk when I'm cooking in large batches, but use my regular 10 in [25 cm] whisk for the basics with great effect.

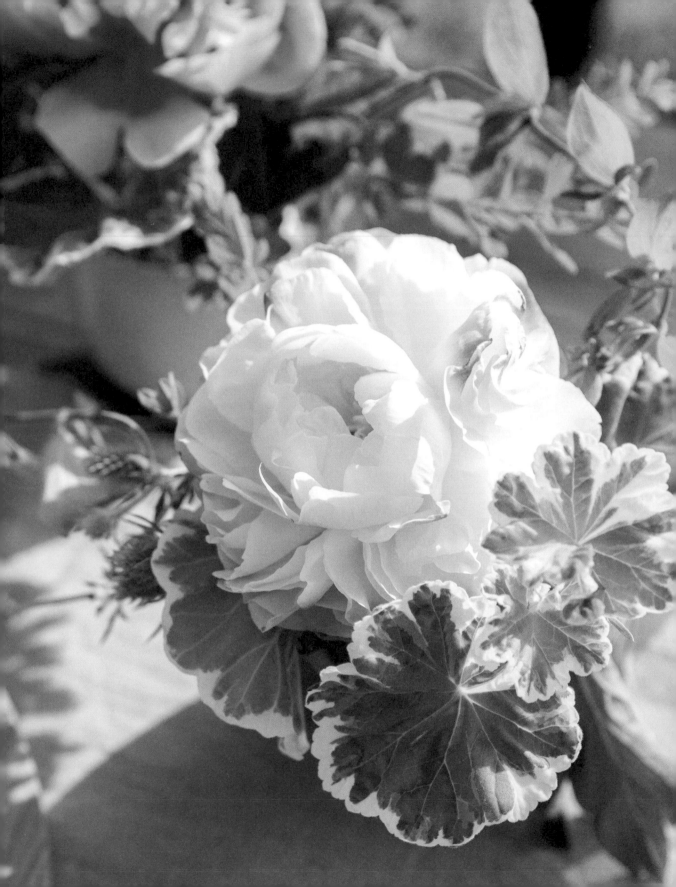

chapter

1

MY BEST BREAKFASTS, HOT DRINKS, AND JUICES

Breakfast is a nonnegotiable in my house. Maybe it's because I wake up really hungry every morning, but I've known forever that I can't function without healthy foods to start my day, and my sons are the same way. This chapter is designed to help you make food that is easy to prepare so you can feel your best every day of the week. Whether you make a batch of the Crustless Mini-Quiches (page 35) on a weekend and reheat them as you're running out the door, or whip up a batch of Strawberry-Basil Smoothies (page 29) on a weekday, making time for sustenance at the beginning of your day will increase your energy, help stabilize your blood sugar and ward off cravings, and help you focus until lunchtime.

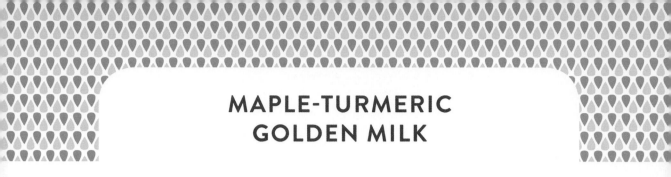

MAPLE-TURMERIC GOLDEN MILK

Ayurvedic medicine has used turmeric for centuries to fight inflammation, colds, arthritis, and even cancer, but it's only recently that the Western world has gone mad for it as well. Take, for example, the "golden milk" craze. This Westernized version of *haldi doodh*, or turmeric milk, which has been served in India for centuries, adds ingredients like cashew milk, coconut oil, and maple syrup to turn it into a decidedly delicious and healthy drink.

In my version, I've added some freshly ground black pepper, as its thermogenic properties increase your metabolic rate while increasing the absorption of the turmeric. (Pretty amazing!) Whip this up and you might just kick your morning coffee habit, or use it as a relaxing drink before bedtime.

PREPARATION TIME
5 minutes

SERVES
1

1 cup [240 ml] unsweetened cashew or almond milk

1 Tbsp maple syrup, plus more as needed

1½ tsp ground turmeric

1½ tsp grated fresh ginger

½ tsp freshly ground black pepper

In a small saucepan over medium heat, combine the ingredients. Increase the heat to medium-high and bring to a boil, whisking occasionally. Let cool slightly, then serve.

TIP: For a frothy latte, transfer the hot mixture to a blender and blend on high for 1 minute.

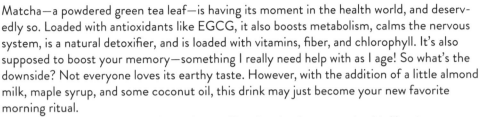

COCONUT-ALMOND MATCHA

Matcha—a powdered green tea leaf—is having its moment in the health world, and deservedly so. Loaded with antioxidants like EGCG, it also boosts metabolism, calms the nervous system, is a natural detoxifier, and is loaded with vitamins, fiber, and chlorophyll. It's also supposed to boost your memory—something I really need help with as I age! So what's the downside? Not everyone loves its earthy taste. However, with the addition of a little almond milk, maple syrup, and some coconut oil, this drink may just become your new favorite morning ritual.

Note: If you've never used matcha, you'll notice that its texture is a bit like cinnamon—it gets lumpy if you add a lot of liquid to it at once. The trick to a frothy, lump-free matcha latte is to whisk the matcha powder with a very small amount of liquid so that it forms a paste before adding more liquid.

PREPARATION TIME
5 minutes

SERVES
1

---

1 Tbsp coconut oil	1 to 2 Tbsp maple syrup
1 cup [240 ml] almond milk	⅛ tsp almond extract (optional)
1 Tbsp green matcha powder	Whipped coconut cream (optional)
	Coconut flakes (optional)

In a small saucepan, melt the coconut oil over very low heat. Add 1 Tbsp of the almond milk and the matcha powder. Whisk until a smooth paste is formed. Slowly whisk in the rest of the almond milk, making sure there are no lumps. Whisk in 1 Tbsp of the maple syrup and the almond extract (if using) and heat over medium heat until barely steaming. Taste and add more maple syrup, as desired.

Top with whipped coconut cream or coconut flakes, if desired. Serve warm.

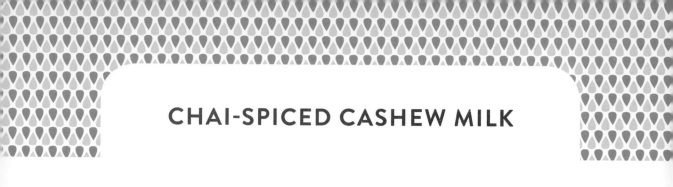

CHAI-SPICED CASHEW MILK

Nut milks are nothing new, but they've become wildly popular as people look for dairy alternatives. I was looking to do something new with cashew milk and my team and I decided to put a chai spin on it. I threw together some spices and bang! Magic happened! The spices add a depth and richness that makes this drink addictive. And you get all the health benefits of the spices, such as increased circulation and better digestion.

If you like the spice blend, you can make a large batch and store it in an airtight container in your pantry for a few months. Add it to your tea, coffee, or even smoothies.

PREPARATION TIME
10 minutes
(plus 20 minutes to soak)

MAKES
8 cups / 2 L

CHAI SPICE BLEND

1 Tbsp ground cinnamon	1½ tsp ground cardamom
1½ tsp ground cloves	½ tsp freshly ground black pepper

CASHEW MILK

2 cups [265 g] unsalted raw cashews	2 Tbsp chai spice blend
8 cups [2 L] purified water	1 Tbsp grated fresh ginger
2 to 4 Tbsp maple syrup	

To make the chai spice blend: Combine all the ingredients in a small bowl and stir. Set aside.

To make the cashew milk: Put the cashews and 4 cups [960 ml] of the water in a blender. Let sit for 20 minutes. Add 2 Tbsp of the maple syrup, the spice blend, and the ginger. Blend at low speed, then slowly increase the speed to high and blend until smooth. Add the remaining 4 cups [960 ml] water and remaining 2 Tbsp of maple syrup (if desired) to reach your preferred consistency and taste.

Store, covered, in the refrigerator for up to 1 week, making sure to stir the milk before serving.

"HAASCAI" BERRY SHAKES
or BOWLS

The acai berry is the ultimate superfood. Loaded with omega fats, protein, and fiber, acai berries also have more antioxidants than blueberries or pomegranates. Grown in the Amazon rainforest, the berries are pureed and frozen to keep their nutritional integrity. Look for organic brands in the supermarket's frozen aisle, as it's the common form sold in the United States. Acai berries have very little natural sugar, so I like to combine them with sweeter fruits like frozen mango, then add a dash of maple syrup. This recipe is delicious as shakes or bowls; the bowls simply use less almond milk.

PREPARATION TIME
10 minutes

SERVES
2

One 3.5 oz [100 g] package frozen acai puree

1 cup [120 g] frozen mango chunks

1 cup [120 q] frozen strawberries

1 to 2 cups [240 to 480 ml] unsweetened almond milk

1 to 2 Tbsp maple syrup

Toppings such as gluten-free granola, toasted sesame or pumpkinseeds, or sliced fruit (for bowls)

Run the acai package under warm water, breaking it into a few pieces so it blends more easily. Cut the package open and put the acai in a blender.

To make shakes: Add the mango, strawberries, 1½ cups [360 ml] of the almond milk, and 1 Tbsp of the maple syrup to the blender. Blend on low speed until the fruit begins to break up, then blend on high speed until smooth. Taste, adding the remaining ½ cup [120 ml] almond milk and remaining 1 Tbsp maple syrup (if desired) to reach your preferred consistency and flavor. Serve immediately.

To make bowls: Add the mango, strawberries, 1 cup [240 ml] of the almond milk, and 2 Tbsp maple syrup to the blender. Blend on low speed until the fruit begins to break up, then blend on high speed until smooth. Taste and add more almond milk as needed to reach the desired consistency. Pour into bowls, add your favorite toppings, and serve.

MEYER LEMON *and* ASIAN PEAR JUICE
with Mint

I love Asian pears. Crisp like an apple, yet sweet like a pear, they have a nuance to their flavor that you don't get from other tree fruits. It's like someone added a hint of maple syrup to them. Because they're so sweet, I like to temper them with the soft acid of Meyer lemons. Meyer lemons are a wonderful source of vitamin C and also contain other anti-oxidants that protect against heart disease and aging in general. Throw in some fresh mint and a little fresh ginger to aid digestion, and it's the perfect drink.

PREPARATION TIME
10 minutes

MAKES
3 cups / 720 ml

SERVES
4

2 lb [910 g] Asian pears

6 Meyer lemons, peeled

¼ cup [5 g] loosely packed fresh mint leaves

One 2 in [5 cm] piece ginger, unpeeled

Wash all the ingredients and pat dry. Cut the pears so they will fit through the juicing chute. Juice the pears, lemons, mint, and ginger according to your juicer's instructions, making sure to pile the mint leaves between pieces of pear, which makes them much easier to juice. Serve immediately.

SOPHIA'S TOASTED ALMOND GRANOLA

with Cardamom and Chocolate Chunks

Sophia Kvochak is a friend and cooking enthusiast. After returning from the holidays, I found this granola on my desk. It was completely addicting, and within the day, I needed to know what was in it. Lucky for me, Sophia was willing to share her recipe.

You can certainly replace the pepitas, dried fruit, or chocolate chunks with your own favorite ingredients, but promise me you'll leave the slivered almonds and cardamom in—together, they're magical.

PREPARATION TIME
10 minutes

COOKING TIME
25 minutes

MAKES ABOUT
7 cups/1.7 L

---

4 cups [400 g] gluten-free rolled oats, such as Bob's Red Mill

1 cup [120 g] slivered almonds

1 cup [120 g] pepitas

1½ tsp ground cinnamon

1 tsp kosher salt

½ tsp ground cardamom

¼ tsp ground ginger

¾ cup [240 ml] maple syrup

½ cup [120 ml] extra-virgin olive oil

1 cup [140 g] dried sour cherries or cranberries

¾ cup [135 g] dark chocolate chunks

Position a rack in the center of the oven and preheat the oven to 350°F [180°C]. Line a baking sheet with parchment paper.

In a large bowl, combine the oats, almonds, pepitas, cinnamon, salt, cardamom, and ginger. Add the maple syrup and oil and stir well. Spread the oat mixture evenly onto the prepared sheet and bake until golden, about 25 minutes, turning the sheet halfway through and stirring with a rubber spatula.

Remove the granola from the oven and let it cool completely. Stir in the dried cherries and chocolate, breaking up any large clumps.

Store in an airtight container for up to 1 month.

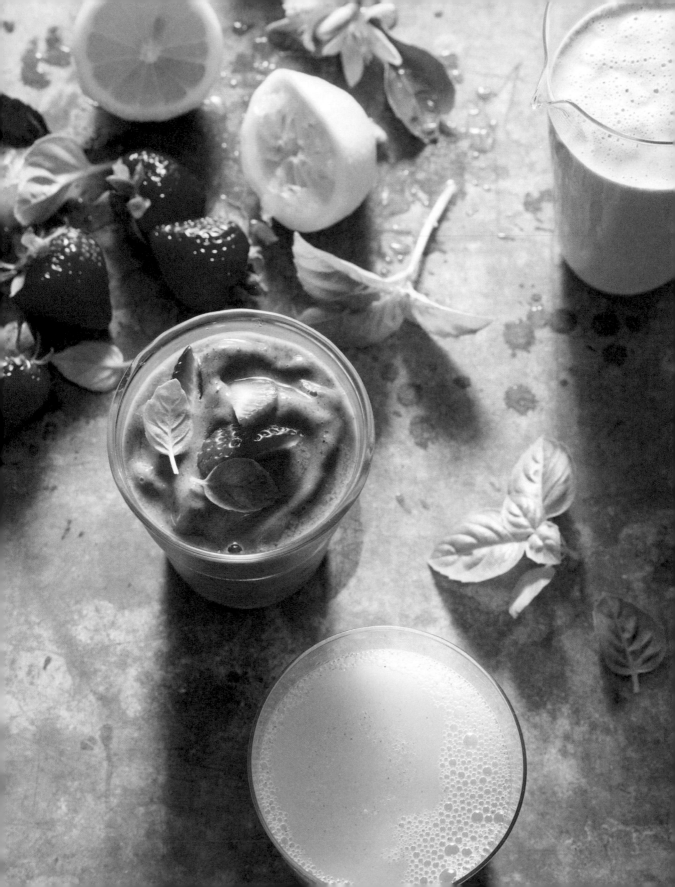

STRAWBERRY-BASIL SMOOTHIES
with Almond Milk and Honey

Strawberries rock. Loaded with vitamin C, folate, potassium, fiber, magnesium, and a ton of other good-for-you things, they aid in brain function and protect against high blood pressure, arthritis, gout, cardiovascular disease, and more. I've always loved the combination of strawberries and basil, and this smoothie is no exception. The basil adds a high note that will start your day off right. (And don't forget, herbs like basil are also loaded with anti-inflammatory and disease-fighting antioxidants.) Who knew a smoothie could taste so good and make you feel so good at the same time?

PREPARATION TIME
5 minutes

MAKES
2 cups / 480 ml

SERVES
2

1 cup [120 g] frozen strawberries

1 cup [240 g] unsweetened almond milk

12 fresh basil leaves

1 Tbsp honey

Combine all the ingredients in a blender. Starting on low speed, puree the mixture until the strawberries begin to break up. Slowly turn the blender speed to high, and puree until there are no lumps, about 1 minute. Serve immediately.

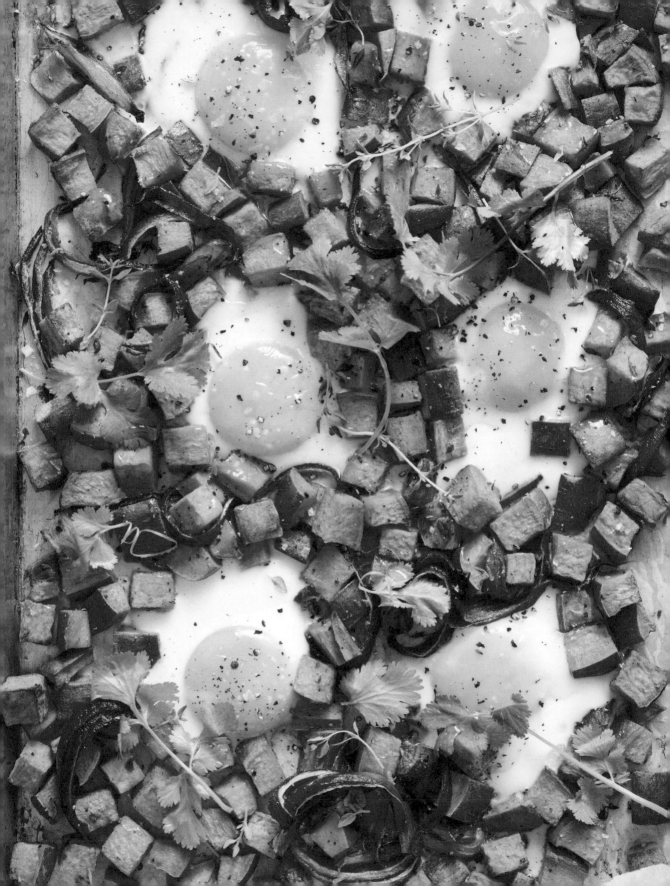

SHEET-PAN SMOKY SWEET POTATO HASH

with Oven-Roasted Eggs

I love savory one-dish breakfasts that fuel me through my mornings at work or at home. Sweet potatoes fill you up and, because their low glycemic index keeps your blood sugar from rising too quickly, they keep you satiated much longer than russet potatoes would. Just be careful not to caramelize them for too long, as that will break down the fiber that works so hard to keep you full. Flavored with alliums and spices and topped with eggs, this may be the easiest, most brilliant savory breakfast around.

PREPARATION TIME
15 minutes

COOKING TIME
35 minutes

SERVES
4

3 large sweet potatoes (about 2 lb [910 g], unpeeled, cut into ½ in [12 mm] dice

1 red onion, cut into ½ in [12 mm] wedges

3 Tbsp extra-virgin olive oil

2 tsp fresh thyme leaves, whole

1 garlic clove, minced

¼ tsp smoked paprika

Kosher salt

Freshly ground pepper

4 eggs

Flaked sea salt

Fresh cilantro leaves

Preheat the oven to 425°F [220°C]. Line a baking sheet with parchment paper or use a nonstick baking sheet.

Combine the sweet potatoes, onion, oil, thyme, garlic, and paprika on the baking sheet and toss to coat. Season generously with kosher salt and pepper. Spread in a single layer. Roast until the potatoes are golden and crisp, about 30 minutes.

Remove the baking sheet from the oven and create four nests in the potatoes. Crack an egg into each nest and sprinkle with kosher salt and pepper. Return to the oven and cook just until the egg whites are set, about 6 minutes, watching closely to ensure the yolks don't cook.

Spoon the eggs and hash onto serving plates, sprinkle with flaked sea salt and cilantro leaves, and serve immediately.

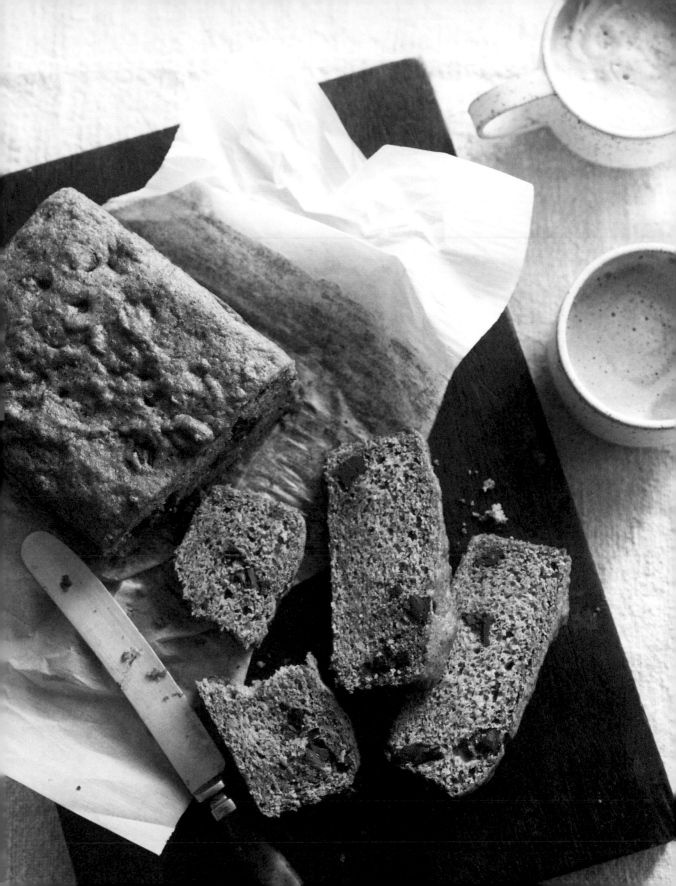

ALMOND FLOUR BANANA BREAD

with Dark Chocolate Chunks

Ever since I stopped eating gluten, I've looked at the pastry counters at my local coffee shops enviably, wishing I could order something every once in a blue moon to dunk in my coffee. Something sweet, dense, and chocolaty, something that really counts. This. Is. It. Think of this ooey, gooey, chocolaty banana bread as a "better for you" version of the usual. Yes, it's got sugar and some refined gluten-free flour, but it also has almond flour and dark chocolate, which means it packs more of a nutritional punch than a typical banana bread. So live a little, and enjoy a slice of this delicious banana bread with a cup of coffee.

PREPARATION TIME	COOKING TIME	SERVES
10 minutes	1 hour	8

2 very ripe bananas, mashed

½ cup [100 g] firmly packed brown sugar

½ cup [120 ml] unsweetened almond milk

¼ cup [40 g] unrefined coconut oil

1 egg

2 tsp vanilla extract

¾ cup [120 g] gluten-free flour, such as Cup4Cup or Bob's Red Mill

¾ cup [90 g] almond flour

2 tsp baking powder

1½ tsp kosher salt

1 tsp ground cinnamon

¾ cup [135 g] dark chocolate chunks

Preheat the oven to 350°F [180°C]. Lightly grease a 9 by 5 in [23 by 13 cm] loaf pan.

In a large mixing bowl, whisk together the bananas, brown sugar, almond milk, coconut oil, egg, and vanilla to combine. In a separate large mixing bowl, whisk together both flours, baking powder, salt, and cinnamon. Whisk the wet ingredients into the dry ingredients until completely incorporated. Gently fold in the chocolate chunks.

Transfer the batter to the prepared loaf pan and bake until a toothpick inserted into the center of the loaf comes out clean, 55 to 60 minutes. Let the bread cool in the pan on a wire rack for 10 minutes, then invert onto the rack and allow to cool for another 30 minutes. Slice and serve.

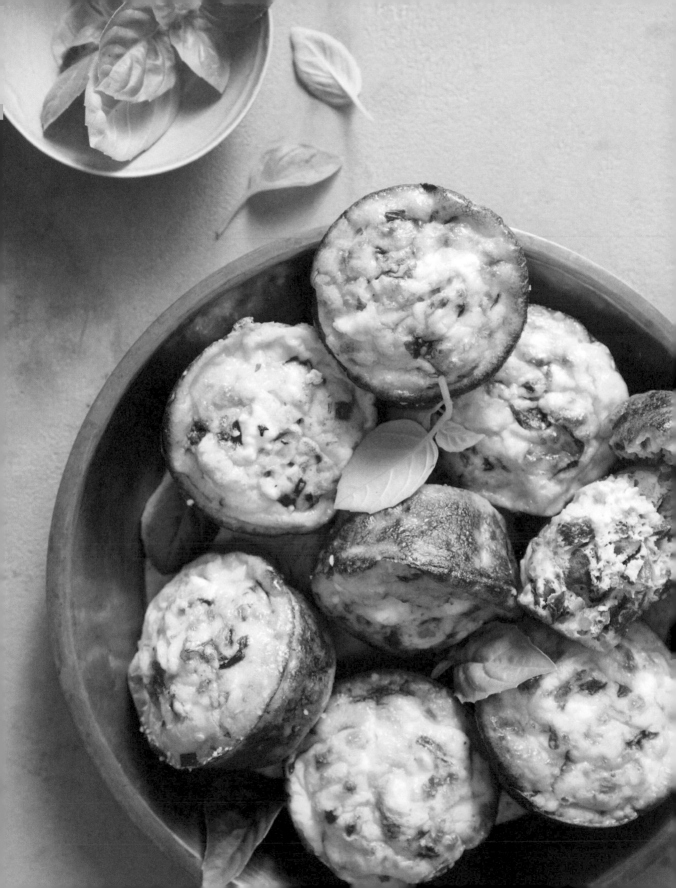

CRUSTLESS MINI-QUICHES

with Roasted Red Pepper, Basil, and Goat Cheese

Still considered by many to be the perfect food, eggs are loaded with protein, vitamins A and B, and biotin. They're also anti-inflammatory superheroes, which we need to look and feel our best! This recipe is a family fave because you can make a batch or two, eat a few right then and there, and then pop the rest in the refrigerator. When you're running out the door in the morning or think you don't have time for breakfast, you can heat one of these up in 30 seconds and give your morning a protein-packed boost.

Use whatever veggies and cheese you like. Spinach and Swiss cheese would be delicious, as would Cheddar and a little bit of leftover roasted broccoli. In this version, I've mixed in some roughly chopped basil for color and an extra punch of nutrition.

PREPARATION TIME
15 minutes

COOKING TIME
20 minutes

MAKES
12 mini-quiches

1 Tbsp extra-virgin olive oil	5 oz [140 g] goat cheese, crumbled
½ yellow onion, finely diced	¼ cup [10 g] chopped fresh basil
10 eggs	Kosher salt
1 roasted red pepper, finely diced	Freshly ground pepper

Preheat the oven to 350°F [180°C]. Spray a 12-cup muffin tin generously with cooking spray.

In a small skillet over medium heat, warm the oil. Add the onion and cook, stirring frequently, until softened, about 7 minutes. Transfer to a small plate to cool.

In a large bowl, whisk the eggs until frothy. Add the cooled onion, red pepper, goat cheese, and basil, and season with salt and pepper. Stir to combine. Divide evenly among the muffin cups. Bake until the eggs have puffed up, are set, and are beginning to brown, 18 to 20 minutes. Serve immediately, or allow to cool on a wire rack, then refrigerate in an airtight container for up to 4 days. Reheat in the microwave for 15 to 20 seconds.

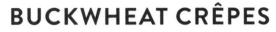

BUCKWHEAT CRÊPES
with Berry Compote and Maple-Whipped Goat Cheese

Don't let the name "buckwheat" fool you: buckwheat is not wheat at all. In fact, it's the seed of a broadleaf plant and is considered a superfood thanks to its ability to stabilize blood sugar, lower cholesterol, and fight inflammation. Luckily for the gluten-free crowd, it can be ground into flour and used as a base for soba noodles and pastas or for this delicious, nutty-tasting crêpe batter. (The French already do this and they look fabulous, so let's be cool and follow suit.) I use a little bit of gluten-free flour to round out the recipe. And the compote on its own is heaven.

PREPARATION TIME
20 minutes

COOKING TIME
30 minutes

SERVES
4

STRAWBERRY-BLUEBERRY COMPOTE

1½ cups [180 g] strawberries, hulled and sliced

1½ cups [180 g] blueberries

3 Tbsp fresh lemon juice

2 tsp maple syrup

¼ tsp ground ginger

Pinch of kosher salt

WHIPPED GOAT CHEESE

8 oz [225 g] goat cheese

2 Tbsp maple syrup

2 Tbsp unsweetened almond milk

Pinch of kosher salt

CRÊPES

2 cups [480 ml] unsweetened almond milk

¾ cup [120 g] gluten-free flour, such as Cup4Cup or Bob's Red Mill

½ cup [60 g] buckwheat flour

3 eggs

¼ tsp kosher salt

Butter or neutral oil for the pan

To make the compote: In a medium saucepan, combine the strawberries, blueberries, lemon juice, syrup, ginger, and salt. Cook over low heat, stirring occasionally, until the berries break down and the sauce thickens, about 20 minutes. Set aside and cover to keep warm.

To make the whipped goat cheese: In the bowl of a stand mixer fitted with the paddle attachment, combine the goat cheese, syrup, almond milk, and salt. Beat on medium-high speed until light and fluffy, about 3 minutes. Set aside.

To make the crêpes: In a blender, process the almond milk, both flours, the eggs, and salt on high speed until combined, about 30 seconds.

In a crêpe pan or small skillet over medium heat, melt 1 tsp butter so that it coats the entire pan. Pour just enough batter into the center of the pan to coat the bottom in a thin layer, tilting the pan to spread the batter around. Cook until the bottom of the crêpe is set, about 2 minutes. Flip the crêpe over and cook an additional 1 to 2 minutes. Transfer to a plate and cover. Repeat with the remaining batter, adding 1 tsp of butter to the pan before each crêpe is made if necessary.

Serve the crêpes with the whipped goat cheese and berry compote.

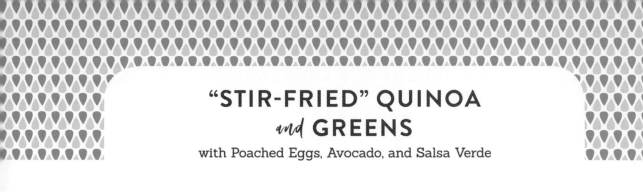

"STIR-FRIED" QUINOA *and* GREENS

with Poached Eggs, Avocado, and Salsa Verde

I am a creature of habit, and this, my friends, is what I like to call my Groundhog Day breakfast. Who can blame me? Breakfast can make or break how you feel for the rest of the day, so I always love to start with something that is going to fill me up and give me energy. With a little leftover quinoa as a base and tons of greens for fiber, protein, and anti-inflammatory properties, this is truly the breakfast of champions. If you make quinoa during the week, make a little extra so you can save it for breakfast. Then add whatever other veggies and aromatics you've got in the fridge. While you're sautéing those ingredients, you can boil some water to poach your eggs. (For my foolproof poached egg technique, see page 232.) I promise, once you master this technique you'll have an amazing breakfast for yourself in 15 minutes or less.

PREPARATION TIME
15 minutes

COOKING TIME
15 minutes

SERVES
4

---

4 Tbsp [60 ml] extra-virgin olive oil

2 shallots, thinly sliced

1 garlic clove, minced or grated

3 cups [600 g] cooked quinoa (page 231)

½ tsp red pepper flakes

1 bunch red chard, stemmed and coarsely chopped

Kosher salt

Freshly ground pepper

4 poached eggs

1 avocado, thinly sliced

¼ cup [60 ml] Preserved Lemon Gremolata (page 221) or other green sauce

Flaked sea salt

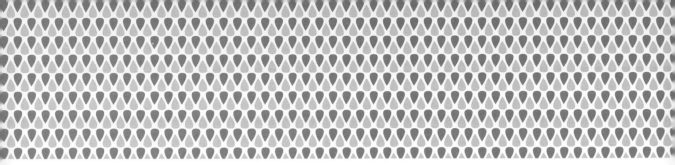

In a large nonstick skillet over medium heat, warm 2 Tbsp of the oil. Add the shallots and cook, stirring frequently, until softened, about 3 minutes. Add the garlic and cook until fragrant, about 1 minute. Add 1 Tbsp oil and increase the heat to medium-high. Stir in the quinoa and cook, stirring infrequently, until the quinoa begins to brown and crisp, about 5 minutes. Transfer to a bowl.

Add the remaining 1 Tbsp oil and the red pepper flakes to the empty pan over medium heat. Add the chard and cook until tender and wilted, about 5 minutes. Toss the chard with the quinoa and season with kosher salt and pepper.

Divide the quinoa and chard among four bowls. Top each with a poached egg, one-quarter of the avocado slices, and a generous spoonful of gremolata. Sprinkle with flaked sea salt and serve immediately.

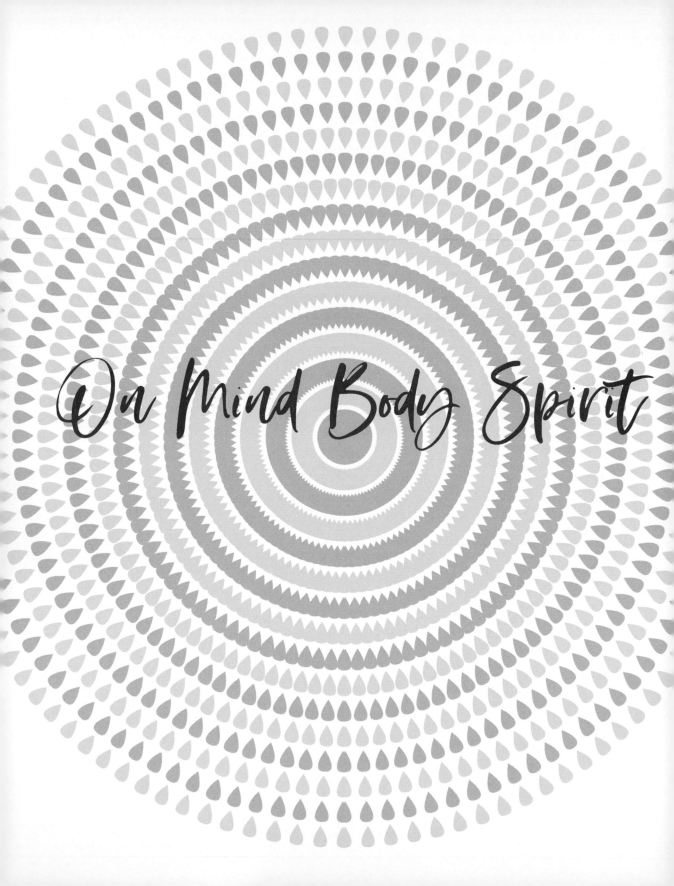

On Mind Body Spirit

The HEALING PROPERTIES of YOGA

with certified yoga instructor Lindsey Valdez

Lindsey Valdez is a longtime friend from the food world. After too many years of the hardcore New York City celebrity chef lifestyle, she found herself burned out and feeling unhealthy. Her true passion was yoga, and her dedication to the practice gave her the faith to quit her enviable job in food publicity and pursue a career in yoga. Now she's a certified yoga and meditation instructor, runs her own private practice, LVLYoga, and teaches in studios across New York and Los Angeles.

As Lindsey was growing her business, we created a ritual where every time I'd go to New York for work, she'd come to my hotel and give me a private lesson. It was a great way to catch up and the perfect way to relieve my aches and pains after a six-hour flight. Our joke was that it was the only time I did yoga! Luckily, Lindsey relocated to Los Angeles, making it more convenient for me to take advantage of her services. Together, Lindsey and I developed a daily yoga practice that's had a huge impact on my well-being.

The results have been remarkable. My aches and pains have been drastically reduced. My lower back started to relax, my joints felt better, and I held less stress in my body. After being unable to walk for two weeks in the spring due to a recurring disk injury, I returned to moving without pain. When I do get stiff after too much driving or flying, my yoga practice can pull me out of it.

Here, Lindsey weighs in about her yoga philosophy and shares a simple, yet life-changing, daily practice.

BENEFITS OF YOGA

I believe one of the most profound yet simple benefits of yoga is the spaciousness gained from the practice. In yoga the *asana*—the Sanskrit word meaning "seat," which refers to the physical yoga postures or poses—creates obvious physical space by lengthening, stretching, and realigning our bodies. But the physical body is only one layer of the practice. Yoga is also meant to help you connect with and penetrate the deeper layers of yourself so that you may gain spaciousness in your energetic, mental, emotional, and spiritual bodies.

Connection is the other invaluable benefit of yoga. Yoga is a self-study practice where we tune IN, rather than zone OUT. In a very tangible way, you connect with yourself through mindful movement of the body. You place your body into shapes, and every pose is guided by the breath with a conscious and purposeful inhale and exhale.

The poses are meant to be experienced through sensations of the body—not the thinking mind. In doing this, we can allow the mind to stop ruminating on thoughts of the past or future or on expectations, and simply try to make a connection with what we feel in the present moment. This is how you know when you've gone too far in a pose, when you can go further in a pose, or when you've found your sweet spot. You'll often hear yoga instructors say that "the body doesn't lie," because it's true, but we must pay attention in order to listen to and understand our bodies. Instead of simply being an "exercise" for the body, yoga offers a holistic approach to wellness and well-being.

Today, yoga is recognized as a clinically viable treatment at major health care centers across the world, including Memorial Sloan Kettering Cancer Center and Harvard Medical School, and there are thousands of articles published in medical journals showing academic research to support the healing benefits of the practice. These include increased circulation, toning and strengthening of the muscles, improved joint health and flexibility, better balance and healthier postural habits, and even increased bone density.

PRANAYAMA, OR BREATHWORK

Prana in Sanskrit translates to "energy" or "life force." From the yogic point of view, everything in the universe that assumes the quality of aliveness is throbbing with prana. When we practice yoga, the *pranayama* refers to the breathwork we are doing as we move through the poses. This is the crucial element of the practice. It *is* yoga—otherwise we'd just be doing another form of exercising or stretching. The breath initiates every pose and measures every pause within the pose. The breath literally guides the practice. I begin all of my yoga classes by cuing my students to settle into stillness in their bodies, and then locate their breath. I find that an accessible way to locate the breath is by touch; placing one hand on the low belly and one hand over the heart helps you feel your body breathing with the rise and fall of the low belly and the chest.

There's a direct relationship between our breath and heart rate, and our sympathetic and parasympathetic nervous systems. For example, if you're feeling panicky or anxious, your body switches into fight-or-flight mode and the sympathetic nervous system kicks in to release the stress hormone cortisol, causing your breath to become short and shallow, and your heart rate to speed up and become rapid or even frantic. To combat this, you can use the pranayama breathwork techniques to stop to ask yourself, "Where did my breath go?" If you take pause to slow down your breathing and start to control your breath again, your heart rate will slow and you will be able to switch back to a "rest and digest" state, with the parasympathetic nervous system balancing you out. Practicing this on and off the mat is how yoga becomes true connection. Steady breathing leads to a steady mind.

LINDSEY'S REJUVENATING DAILY YOGA PRACTICE

I chose this sequence with the intention to make it accessible for anyone because I truly believe that yoga is for everyone. All you need is a yoga mat. I wanted it to be approachable, and above all I wanted it to feel good. I also wanted the practice to be suitable for any time of day, so there could be no excuses for procrastination or avoidance. These poses are great for your morning rise-and-shine routine, and they work just as well before bedtime, too. This practice is created for all levels of practitioners, and is safe for pregnant women, aging adults, and even children.

The benefits of this sequence include the meditative pranayama breathwork practice, joint care, back care, detoxification, strengthening and lengthening of the muscles, heart opening, and of course constructive rest and relaxation. My hope is that this practice not only stretches and strengthens your body, but also your mind and heart, ultimately leading you to fall in love with your yoga practice, as I have with mine!

RECLINED BOUND ANGLE POSE

This pose helps release spinal tension as well as open the hips. This shape is accessible to all levels of practitioners and allows for simultaneous grounding as well as opening of the body, mind, and heart.

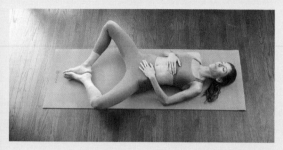

- Begin on your back. Bring the soles of your feet together to touch and allow your knees to fall apart, creating space in your hips.

- Place your right hand on your low belly and your left hand over your heart. Softly close your eyes and mouth as you relax your entire body.

PRANAYAMA BREATHWORK:

- Begin to notice and feel your body breathing. As you inhale, feel your low belly expand under your right hand. As you exhale, feel your belly fall. Repeat three rounds of breath, inhaling and exhaling through your nose. Aim to keep your mouth closed.

- Now begin to control your breath by taking deeper, more expansive breaths in through your nose as you lengthen your inhale from your low belly hand and draw it up into your heart, feeling your ribs expand and your chest rise up under your left hand. Exhale through your nose, and feel your chest drop, your ribs contract, and your low belly fall beneath your right hand. Repeat three to five more cycles of this conscious breath. We call this *ujjayi* breath, which has an audible sound as it passes over the back of the throat.

INTENTION SETTING:

- Softly slide your right hand over your left hand and take a moment to set a clear and positive intention or dedication for your practice. This will infuse your practice with purpose.

- Open your eyes and bring your knees together, and place your feet flat on the mat with your legs bent.

SUPINE TWIST

This pose lengthens the spine and allows for a gentle twist of the abdomen, cleansing the digestive system.

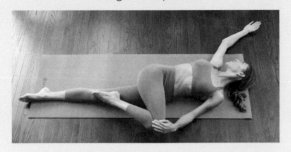

- From your finishing position of the last pose, hug your right knee into your chest as you extend your left leg long away from you.

- Take your right leg across to the left side of your body, twisting your torso. Extend your right arm and turn your head and neck over your right shoulder to deepen the twist.

- Stay in the pose, breathing your ujjayi pranayama for three to five cycles. Then come back to center and extend your right leg straight on the mat.

- Hug your left knee to your chest and repeat the twist on the other side.

CAT/COW

Cat/Cow opens the front and back of the body, as well as the wrist and shoulder joints, and prepares the spine for movement. It also pumps oxygen in and out of the body, creating better flow of prana.

COME TO TABLETOP POSITION:

On all fours, stack your shoulders over your wrists with your hands shoulder-distance apart and your fingers and palms spread wide. Stack your hips over your knees with your knees hip-distance apart.

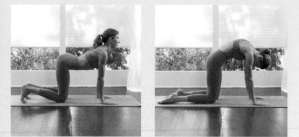

COW:

- Inhale, drop your belly as you lift your chin, opening the throat space and widening your collarbones as you lift your tailbone and hips.

CAT:

- Exhale and round your back, pulling your belly in toward your spine, tucking your chin to your chest, and closing the throat as you push the mat away.

- Repeat two more times.

CHILD'S POSE

This modified version of Child's Pose creates openness in the shoulders and helps flush out the intercostal muscles, which are the breathing muscles between our ribs. It helps us tune back into our body and breath and refocus.

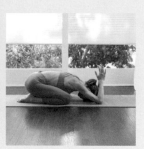

- From tabletop position, bring your big toes together to touch and your knees wide apart as you sit your hips back and down on your heels, and lay your torso between your thighs.

- Rest your forehead on the mat and touch your palms together in prayer hands (Anjali mudra) above your head. Reach your elbows forward away from the crown of your head and reach your fingers and thumbs back toward your seat.

- Remain here for two or three breaths, allowing this posture to be a constructive rest while you breathe deeply and return to your intention or dedication as a reminder of your purpose for practice.

OPPOSITE ARM, OPPOSITE LEG

This pose tones the core and low back muscles and helps develop balance. It's also mental exercise, as it simultaneously engages opposite sides of the body.

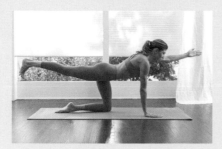

- Return to tabletop position. Extend your right leg backward, keeping your hips square by rotating your right thigh bone toward your left thigh.

- Reach your left arm forward, keeping your arm in line with your shoulder.

- Find your balance point as you hug your right side body and left side body together toward your midline (imagine you're squeezing a block between your thighs to hug your inner thighs toward each other, stabilizing your pelvis). Engage your core by pulling your belly back toward your spine to support your low back.

- Repeat three times on each side, inhaling as you extend and lengthen your spine, and exhaling as you contract and round your spine.

DOWNWARD-FACING DOG

Downward-Facing Dog strengthens the biceps, triceps, and major joints of the arms and wrists. It lengthens and tones the back and legs, and calms the nervous system.

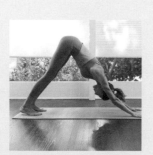

- From tabletop position, tuck your toes under and straighten your legs as best you can while bringing your heels toward the mat. Lift your hips and sit bones up toward the sky as you lengthen the crown of your head down toward the earth.

- Reach your heart toward your thighs as you draw your belly back toward your spine and press your hands down into the mat. Wrap your shoulders down your back and away from your ears to keep length in your neck and upper back.

- Hold and breathe deeply for three to five cycles of ujjayi breath.

PLANK POSE TO LOW PUSH-UP TO COBRA

The following sequence of poses is called a "Vinyasa," meaning a progression of poses linked to create flow. This short sequence heats and energizes the body, and strengthens the entire spinal column and major joints.

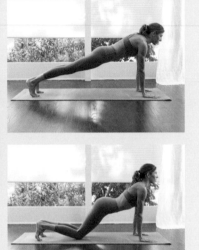

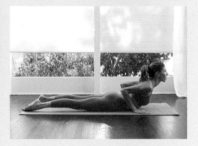

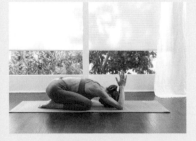

- From Downward-Facing Dog, inhale as you bring your shoulders over your wrists, keeping your body straight and engaging your thighs and core.

- Reach your heels backward as you extend your head and neck forward and lengthen your spine into Plank Pose.

- Exhale, drop your knees to the mat, and bend your elbows as you keep your body straight. Lower your chest with control as you come onto your belly in a Modified Low Push-Up.

- Adjust your hands to ensure they are under your shoulders and bring your legs together, pointing your toes.

- Inhale as you push the tops of your feet into the ground, lifting and curling your upper body and heart off of the mat, engaging your back muscles and leg muscles as you widen through your collarbones and lengthen through your spine.

- Gaze forward or upward as you relax your shoulders down away from your ears and deepen your breath, massaging your low belly into the mat. This is Cobra pose.

- Exhale and push your hips back into Child's Pose.

- Repeat this sequence two more times, finding your moving meditation in the flow.

SUN BREATHS

Sun Breaths are a variation of Sun Salutations, which are a wonderful way to heat the body and burn away tension, stiffness, and soreness through rhythmic breath and fluid movements. This series works the major muscles groups and helps balance the endocrine system and bring mental clarity.

STANDING FORWARD FOLD:

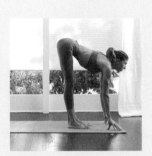

- This standing fold stretches the hamstrings and alleviates lower back pain. It also grounds and calms the nervous system.

- From Child's Pose, come to Downward-Facing Dog and walk your feet forward toward your hands until you arrive at the top of your mat with your feet hip-distance apart, coming into a Forward Fold.

- Exhale deeply as you hinge from your hips and ground your hands onto the mat. Engage your thighs and draw your chest toward your legs. You can keep a soft bend in your knees if necessary.

FLAT BACK:

- This pose stretches the hamstrings and helps alleviate lower back pain. It also strengthens and engages your core and low back muscles, and it encourages deeper breath and circulation of prana.

- From your Forward Fold, inhale and extend your spine by reaching your heart and crown of your head forward, lengthening your spine and the back of your neck.

- Pull your navel in toward your spine as you engage your quadriceps and press your hands into your shins to create more leverage and extension.

- Exhale as you return to Forward Fold.

MOUNTAIN POSE:

- Inhale as you press through the soles of your feet and lift up through your quadriceps and front of the core.

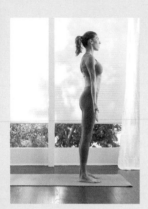

- Reach your arms out and up overhead as you rise up to stand tall.

- Draw your hands together in prayer hands over your heart space.

- As you stand in the pose, make sure your head is over your shoulders, shoulders over your hips, hips over your knees, and knees over your ankles.

- Ground down through your feet and extend up through the crown of your head, standing your tallest as you breathe deeply.

- Tune back into the intention or dedication you made at the beginning of your practice as you center and ground yourself.

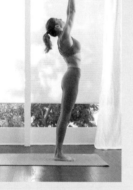

UPWARD SUN SALUTE:

- Inhale and reach your arms up over your head, lengthening your arms and torso.

- Exhale as you swan dive with open arms, hinging at the waist and returning to Forward Fold to start your next round of Sun Breaths.

- Repeat at least two more rounds of Sun Breaths as a moving meditation.

CORPSE POSE

Corpse Pose, or Shavasana, comes at the end of every practice, and it is the most important of all of the asana poses! It allows for all of the previous poses in your practice to be absorbed. It calms the nervous system and releases tension, allowing you to take some precious time out for yourself to truly rest and relax.

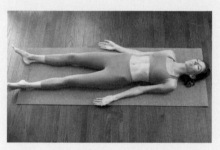

- Come to lie flat on your back, extending your legs long with your feet wider than hip-distance apart.

- Release your arms long down by your sides, away from your body, with your palms facing up in a gesture of openness and receptivity.

- Close your eyes softly as you settle into stillness and relax your entire body as well as your thinking mind.

- Let go of your ujjayi breath and allow your body to go back to breathing naturally. Allow your breath to become calm, neutral, and effortless.

- Try to keep your mind free of thoughts or distractions. Relax and remain here for a minimum of two minutes, preferably five.

- When you are ready, keeping your eyes closed, begin to inhale and exhale deeply again.

- Slowly move your fingers and toes and circle your ankles and wrists, waking yourself up gently.

- Bring both hands to your heart in prayer hands and recall your intention for your practice and seal it in gratitude.

- Know that it takes great courage, discipline, and self-love to come onto your mat to practice, so take a moment to honor yourself and thank yourself for showing up for yourself in this way.

INGREDIENTS *for* LONGEVITY

with nutritionist Rebecca Katz, MS

Rebecca Katz is the one who inspired me to dedicate an entire chapter in this book to greens. I'm so grateful to her as a teacher, and knew I had to interview her so I could share some of her impressive nutritional knowledge with you, too.

Let me tell you a little about Rebecca: She's the founder of the Healing Kitchens Institute, chef emeritus for the Center for Mind-Body Medicine's Food as Medicine professional training, and expert on the role of food in supporting optimal health. Her daily work is directly affecting the landscape of our well-being. She has an MS in health and nutrition education, trained at New York's Natural Gourmet Institute for Health and Culinary Arts, and is the author of five books on nutritional healing, including *The Longevity Kitchen: Satisfying, Big-Flavor Recipes Featuring the Top 16 Age-Busting Power Foods.*

With all of her credentials, I only have one title for her: my Culinary Unicorn! Rebecca translates complicated nutritional facts using relatable metaphors and analogies that stick with you. For instance, she describes our taste buds carrying flavors to the back of our throat as a magic carpet. Lovely, right? Her knowledge is seemingly endless, so it was hard to decide the best way to channel her incredible brain. In the end, we focused on her understanding of ingredients and the foods we need to be eating as we age.

Amanda Haas: What's your take on our attitudes around eating well?

Rebecca Katz: When it comes to food, I believe we can all cut ourselves a big break. Small changes go a long way. I give lots of advice, but I take a nondogmatic approach. It's important to remember that we're all different at different ages. My fifty-six could be your forty-six. The big message I try to convey is that no matter what age you are, you can make a change! You can begin eating better and healing at any time.

Women between the ages of thirty and seventy are expected to do so much for so many people that we forget to take time to prioritize ourselves and our well-being. We all want to be perfect! But nourishing

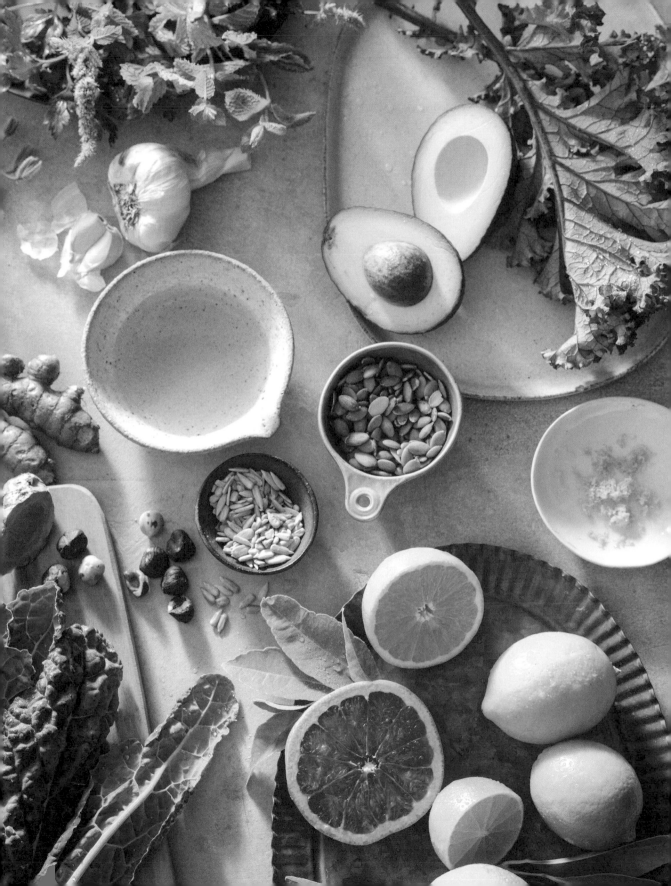

yourself with good food is not about being perfect. You don't have to be a chef. You can take shortcuts, or be an assembler of ingredients instead of a cook, and still incorporate fortifying foods and simple cooking techniques into your daily routine.

When you become empowered by food, you can make a change. There's always an opportunity to feel better. Even if you're in crisis, you can find that pocket of time to cook, if only to cut open an avocado. Cooking is one thing in your life you can control, and this holds true whether you're a gourmet cook or an assembler.

I also think of this middle third of our lives as a fragile time for women. We have to think about the ingredients our bodies really need in order to improve with time. The choices we make now will affect us as we continue to age.

AH: **Why are vegetables so important in our diet?**

RK: It's common knowledge that protein is important, but people get confused about vegetables.

We get the majority of our best vitamins and nutrients through plants, so they should be represented on our plates accordingly. I like to treat my protein as the garnish and the veggies as the main course.

When people say, "Should I steam my veggies or roast them? Can I sauté them or do I need to eat them raw?" I say this: "Roast. Broil. Sauté. Eat them raw!" As a nutritionist, I don't care. Go with whatever preparation is appealing to you. Any way you eat your vegetables, they are immune-boosting and cancer-preventing.

AH: **What ingredients should we focus on as we age, and why?**

RK: First and foremost, healthy fats such as olive oil, avocados, nuts, and seeds.

Avocados are wonder foods because of their fat and fiber content. A lot of people think fiber tastes like cardboard—like bran cereal—but in an avocado, it's voluptuous. One half of an avocado has ten grams of fiber! They're also high in oleic acid, which helps lower cholesterol, and high in complex carbohydrates, so they're incredibly satiating. They also help moderate levels of cortisol, the hormone that can cause weight gain, joint pain, hair loss, and more. The brain is 60 percent fat, and in order to function well and maintain clarity, we need to feed it what it wants!

And olive oil is my absolute favorite food to talk about. I could drink it or put it in an IV drip! A 2017 study conducted at Temple University found that extra-virgin olive oil protects against cognitive decline. The research shows that consumption of extra-virgin olive oil actually protects memory and enhances learning ability. The researchers also discovered that it reduced the formation of amyloid-beta plaques and neurofibrillary tangles in the brain—both of which are markers of Alzheimer's disease. Pretty amazing, right?

Additionally, the fat in olive oil allows your body to absorb the fat-soluble vitamins A, D, E, and K that are in all of those diverse veggies you're eating. Fat also carries taste and flavor, so your broccoli or kale will taste a heck of a lot more exciting when doused in a little olive oil before you roast it. In my experience, olive oil truly transforms the flavor of foods.

AH: **What's the deal when people say if you heat up olive oil too much, you'll create free radicals and ruin all of the positive benefits of it?**

RK: When people say you can't heat olive oil because you create free radicals, I say, "Well, what's worse? Heating up olive oil or not eating it at all?"

It takes a lot of heat to create free radicals. If you're working on a restaurant stove where your pan hits 500°F (260°C) in a matter of seconds, that's one thing. But at home, if you want to get the most nutritional value out of your olive oil, simply heat the pan first, then quickly add the olive oil and immediately add your greens.

Go ahead and roast or sauté your vegetables in olive oil—don't worry about it!

AH: **I know you love cooking with herbs for flavor—we both do—but what about the health benefits of doing this?**

RK: Many of my clients find using herbs and spices in their cooking intimidating. Well, I'm here to show them otherwise. Herbs have concentrated amount of phytochemicals, so, bite per bite, eating food seasoned with herbs is like eating a whole pile of kale! Herbs and spices pack an incredible health punch.

My two favorite herbs are mint and parsley. From a culinary perspective, mint is a rock star. The flavor is so recognizable. It adds a delicious punch in savory foods like salsas, green sauces, or vinaigrettes; it also balances out the sweet notes of chocolate or fruit. From a health perspective, mint is a powerful antioxidant that's been shown to aid digestion; improve nasal health, dental health, and blood circulation; treat dizziness; and even help prevent dandruff. It has so many phytochemicals and is great for your mind and your body. It's also cancer-fighting and a brain booster. Smell it and you'll know—it has a bright, high note that makes food sing.

Parsley is a true unsung hero. It does everything from boosting bone strength to helping bad breath, reducing inflammation in the body, and improving joint pain associated with arthritis, fibromyalgia, and more. It also boosts your immunity. The nutrients in parsley are absorbed so well that you need less of it to have the same positive effect as other greens. Because of its adaptable flavor and incredible health benefits, I love using parsley as a base for all green sauces. It's neutral enough, yet pairs with practically any other herb, like basil, thyme, rosemary, or mint.

For a really easy sauce, chop up some mint and parsley and pour in a little olive oil, a squeeze of lemon juice, salt, and pepper. Go buy a roast chicken and put a little dollop of that sauce on it. It's mind-blowing!

AH: **And what about spices? They've become a staple in my anti-inflammatory cooking.**

RK: When it comes to spices, it's hard to choose! Here are a few I love and why:

Ginger: How I love this spice; let me count the ways. It has anti-inflammatory effects; plus, mothers, grandmothers, aunties, and healers all over the world have turned to ginger for generations to soothe nausea and tummy aches. This rhizome can also decrease pain related to arthritis. Ginger is an antioxidant powerhouse, especially in the area of brain health, where it's been shown to treat memory loss and dementia. Many women experience a loss of mental sharpness as they get into middle age, but ginger has been shown to help prevent that from happening. A study on postmenopausal women revealed that ginger boosted their memory and ability to focus.

Cumin: I call this the quicker-picker-upper spice! It supports digestion and neutralizes the carcinogens our body absorbs. Cumin also improves the body's ability to absorb antioxidants (known as antioxidant efficiency). And it's a source of calcium and magnesium, a pair of minerals that may help prevent cognitive decline.

Cinnamon: This spice is so accessible! It has anti-inflammatory properties and is super high in antioxidants. One teaspoon of cinnamon has the same antioxidant punch as one cup of blueberries. You can't beat that. Cinnamon is particularly good for regulating blood sugar. It also works as a digestive aid, since it stimulates the production of digestive enzymes.

Cayenne: This spice and the rest of the chile pepper family contain capsaicin, which may control certain types of pain. Capsaicin can also trick the body into feeling fuller—the spicy taste stimulates the brain's satiation receptors, triggering the same appetite-suppressing hormones that the stomach naturally sends out when it's full. Capsaicin may also fire up your brain with a boost in cognitive functioning.

Turmeric: The substance that gives turmeric its unique yellow-orange color is called curcumin, which is known for its anti-inflammatory properties. It also aids cognitive functioning and focus.

Turmeric is most absorbable if it's paired with cracked black pepper. I use this spice in curries, and also like to sneak some into my scrambled eggs and salad dressings.

Garlic: It's no wonder that garlic is one of the world's oldest and most cultivated plants—it's a boon to our overall health. It's been shown to boost memory and keep our brains sharp in later life. It's antiviral and antimicrobial, and wonderful to eat when you feel like your immune system needs a boost. Garlic may also help prevent certain yeast infections and is considered a cancer-fighting food.

Garlic contains a number of sulfur compounds, including allicin, which can help prevent free radical damage to the lining of the blood vessels. This limits inflammation, which may help ward off heart attacks and stroke. To access the all-powerful allicin, smash a clove of garlic and allow it to sit for ten minutes before consuming or using it in your cooking.

AH: **Why are you such a fan of eating all greens found in nature?**

RK: Because they are so loaded with nutrients and inflammation-fighting properties, it is literally impossible to eat too many greens in your diet. They are high in all-important vitamins, minerals, and phytochemicals. Whether you like broccoli, arugula, Brussels sprouts, or romaine lettuce, adding green veggies to your diet is a wonderful idea! Eating cruciferous green vegetables is like taking a broom and cleaning out your system. They're high in insoluble fiber, which enhances the process of elimination—hence the analogy of the broom!

AH: **We share a special love for citrus, so I'm interested to hear what you think of its health benefits.**

RK: I joke that I moved to California for the Meyer lemons! You know that I love all citrus fruits, both for their flavor and because they're another example of Mother Nature's healing magic. Consuming citrus can help ward off colds, satiate you with fiber, flush excess sodium from your body, improve your heart health, and help you maintain a healthy body weight. That's just the beginning.

So often we use the juice from the citrus or simply eat the flesh, but don't forget that there are health benefits to all parts of the fruit. When you cook with preserved lemons, you're using the skin of the lemon as well, increasing the health benefits. Or if you grate the zest into a recipe, you capture all of the healthy oils from the peel, which can help prevent skin cancer and diabetes and promote good cholesterol.

Try to zest, preserve, or eat the peel whenever possible. I like to use a Microplane and add zest to salad dressings, sauces (especially pesto), and sautéed vegetables. Using the zest is a great way to add a bright note to your cooking without adding more acid. Take advantage of all parts of lemons, limes, oranges, blood oranges, and grapefruit. (Be mindful that grapefruit contains compounds that can amplify the effect of certain medications, so be sure to speak to your doctor about eating grapefruit if you are taking any medication.)

AH: **Rebecca, after you shared all of your wisdom with me, you inspired me to make these foods an even larger part of my life! Any last words of wisdom for someone looking to improve how they eat?**

RK: Turn your black-and-white food world into Technicolor! A plate full of color means you are loading up on the important phytonutrients that can work better than anything else on the planet to balance your immune system, reduce inflammation, and make you feel better at any age.

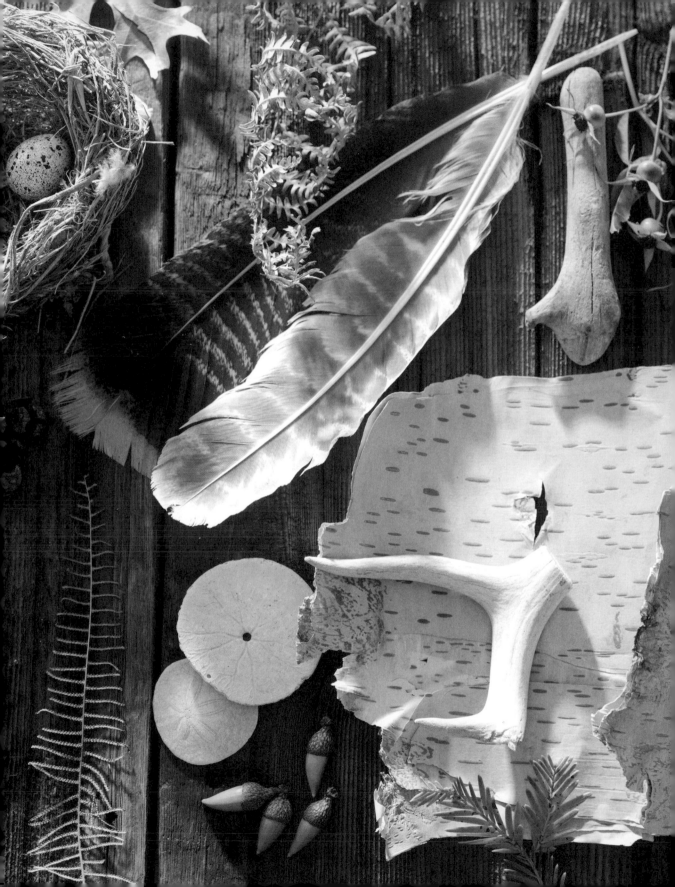

TIME *in* NATURE

As a suburban dweller and urban worker, I can go for weeks without real time out-doors, especially in the winter when it rains. I might sneak out for a walk with a friend over the weekend or play basketball outside with my boys for thirty minutes, but over the last few years, I've noticed that our collective obsession with screen time has contributed to me spending less time in nature. Even as I've consciously tried to increase my time outside, I've found social media distracting me.

Turns out I'm not the only person trading time outdoors for screen time. In March of 2017, TechCrunch reported that adults are spending an average of five hours a day on mobile apps. That doesn't even include time watching regular tele-vision. And Common Sense Media reported that teenagers are now spending an average of *nine* hours a day consuming media. The numbers are staggering, and I can't help but recognize the generational shift from my summer days as a kid swim-ming all day and riding my bike around the neighborhood at night to my sons begging to have their friends over or to hang out so they can play the hottest new video game. Honestly, I'm just as bad. I find myself checking Instagram and texts constantly, at least every few minutes, unless I put my phone away.

I don't want this to be our norm. What I really crave is time in nature away from a screen. By "nature," I mean big trees or expansive views: no buildings, no phone or laptop, no distractions except the sound of the wind and the beautiful scenery. I mean time at the ocean when you can just walk and get lost in the whoosh of the waves as they crash on the shore, their quiet retreat, and rhythmic repeat.

One summer I took my kids to San Diego, and my son Connor and I boogie-boarded together for the first time. As I treaded water in the freezing Pacific—65°F [18°C] on a warm day—I looked over and saw Connor looking the happiest I'd seen him in years. And I felt better than I had in weeks. The waves were pounding us, we were shivering, yet we kept laughing and going back for more.

Connecting with nature brings us real happiness. A study published in the jour-nal *Scientific Reports* shows that the sounds of nature—anything from leaves rustling in the wind to water splashing on river rocks—can bring us to a relaxed state. What's the scientific explanation for the positive effects on our psyche? The sounds physi-cally alter the connections in our brains, reducing our body's fight-or-flight instinct. Fascinating! As I dug into the positive benefits of a little time in nature, the list grew and grew. Here are a few.

RESTORES MENTAL ENERGY

You know that feeling you get when you simply cannot think anymore? I call it brain fatigue. The *Journal of Environmental Psychology* reported that spending time in the great outdoors creates a sense of awe, a surefire way to get a mental boost. Even looking at pictures of nature proved beneficial for some people's mental energy levels (although I think seeing the Grand Canyon in person is a bit more awe-inspiring than seeing a photo!). Time in nature can also aid in concentration and sharpen our thinking.

REDUCES STRESS

The *Scandinavian Journal of Forest Research* discovered that children who spent two nights in the forest showed reduced levels of cortisol, the hormone that marks stress in our bodies, compared to children who spent the same amount of time in a city. An overnight stay isn't even necessary to reap some of the benefits. Another study showed that cortisol levels and heart rates were both lower in people who spend time among trees and nature instead of in a constant city environment. (Forest therapy is a real thing!) And even employees with a view of nature from their desks report lower stress and higher job satisfaction.

IMPROVES MENTAL HEALTH

Studies published in *Environmental Science and Technology* and the *Journal of Affective Disorders* have shown that exercising in nature—even walking—can improve moods and self-esteem and decrease anxiety, and is a clinically useful supplemental treatment for major depressive disorder.

It's natural magic! Making a little time for nature—a hike in nearby woods, a twenty-four-hour escape to the mountains, a weekend camping trip, or a visit to the ocean—can improve your mood and outlook. Reduced stress increases our life span. Nature is medicine.

MASSAGE THERAPY *for* SELF-CARE

I'm a huge believer in massage for my well-being. After struggling with two back injuries for most of my life, I've found it to be really beneficial in reducing muscle tension and fatigue. I know that having regular massages can seem like a luxury rather than a necessity. But massage is finally hitting the mainstream as a healing practice. Many employers allow you to pay for massage therapy out of your flexible spending account, much like acupuncture and other important alternative therapies.

Besides being incredibly relaxing and mood-enhancing, massage therapy has been proven in studies to reduce stress, pain, and muscle tension. It has also become a useful tool to help relieve anxiety, digestive disorders, fibromyalgia, joint pain, insomnia, headaches, and many sports-related injuries.

There are many different types of massage, so you'll want to try a few and see what feels best for you. I choose what type of massage to get depending on how I'm feeling. If I have a lot of muscle tension or have been in spasm, I lean toward deep tissue or hot stone massage. When I simply want to relax and let go of stress, I prefer Swedish or aromatherapy massage. Many massage therapists are trained in more than one type of practice, so if you describe what you're looking to get out of the massage (for example, pain relief, relaxation, or muscle tension relief), they will often make a suggestion. Here are a few common techniques.

SWEDISH MASSAGE

The most common form of massage in the United States, Swedish massage is gentle and relaxing. It uses long smooth strokes, usually with oil or lotion, to manipulate superficial layers of muscle. Based on Western concepts of anatomy and physiology, Swedish massage is good for stress relief, relaxation, and improved circulation.

AROMATHERAPY MASSAGE

Aromatherapy massage incorporates essential oils to aid relaxation and address specific health needs or problems. The essential oils are used in the massage and breathed in through the nose, stimulating smell receptors, which then send messages through the nervous system to the limbic system, the part of the brain that controls emotions. Aromatherapy can be used to reduce stress and anxiety, combat depression, ease headaches, and even alleviate PMS for some.

There are many different essential oils to choose from for aromatherapy; some are known for their calming properties and others are known for energizing properties. For example, lavender oil is often used to treat stress, anxiety, depression, and insomnia, while peppermint oil is used as a natural decongestant. Talk to your massage therapist about which oils might be the best fit for your needs.

HOT STONE MASSAGE

In this style of massage, smooth, heated stones are used on specific points of the body and to perform the massage itself. Heat from the stones eases muscle tension and pain by increasing blood flow. When my back has been in complete spasm, I have had tremendous results from hot stone massage. You should always consult a doctor when treating injuries, but I have found a few practitioners who have been able to relieve my pain significantly through this type of massage.

DEEP TISSUE MASSAGE

During deep tissue massage, deep pressure is applied to problem areas using forceful strokes. The intense pressure reaches deeper layers of muscle and connective tissue than traditional massage. It is beneficial in relieving chronic muscle tension. It can be painful, so it's important to communicate with your massage therapist about the level of pressure you prefer, and check with your doctor to make sure this treatment is safe for you.

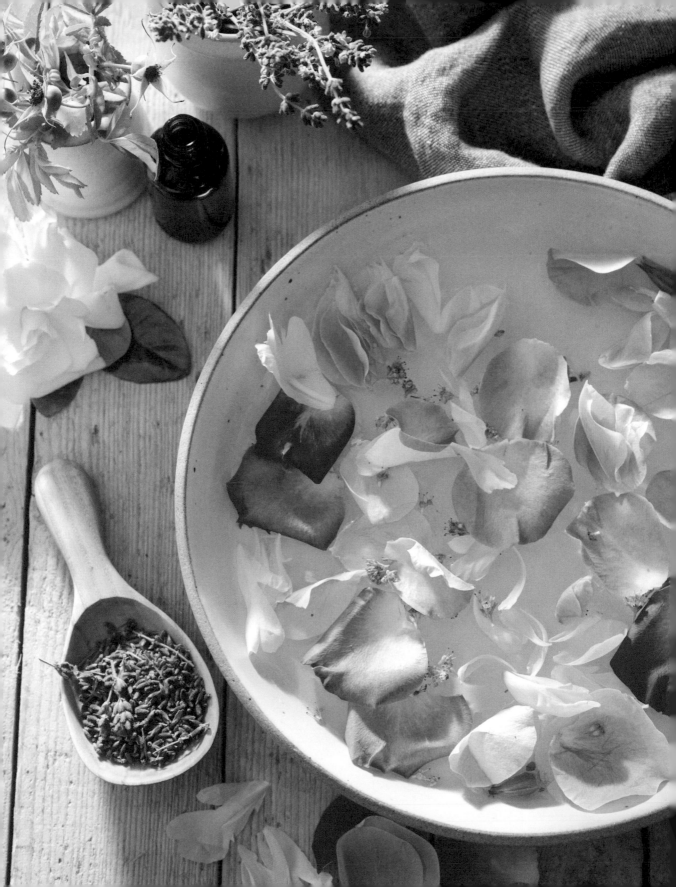

SHIATSU MASSAGE

With roots in Chinese medicine, this form of massage is energy-centric. Without use of oil or lotion, acupressure points are stimulated in a rhythmic sequence along the body. The goal of shiatsu massage is to restore proper patterns of energy flow (also known as *qi*).

The body's qi travels throughout the body like a system of rivers and streams. In certain defined pathways known as meridians, qi flows in a more concentrated manner. When the body experiences tension and stress caused by excess energy, or weakness or emptiness caused by too little energy, qi can become blocked or stagnant.

Your practitioner will identify where the qi is blocked and apply pressure on the proper meridians. They may also use rocking, stretching, and joint rotations to help release the excess energy. Although viewed as "alternative" by many people in America, to the Chinese, shiatsu is considered a complementary treatment to Western medicine, and is believed to reduce anxiety and depression, and improve muscle tension and tension headaches.

THAI MASSAGE

Also known as Thai yoga massage, this style is a combination of acupressure, Indian Ayurvedic principles, and assisted yoga postures that aims to align the body's energy. It is performed fully clothed and there is constant contact between the therapist and the recipient. Instead of rubbing the muscles, the body is rocked, stretched, compressed, and pulled. Instead of lying passively while the massage therapist works on your body, it is a very active form of therapy. A traditional Thai massage can last up to two hours, as the practitioner works the entire body to align energy, which can release tension and improve blood flow to all areas of the body.

REFLEXOLOGY

One of my personal favorites, reflexology is performed primarily on the feet. A reflexologist uses acupressure on certain points on the feet—and sometimes the hands—to relax and improve other points in the body. The premise is that there are reflex areas on the feet that correspond to other parts of the body, so if there is a blockage of qi in a specific part of the body like the liver, heart, or even the neck, acupressure on the correlating area on the foot will improve the well-being of the related part of the body.

There has been little evidence in Western medicine that reflexology has any proven benefits for medical conditions; however, people who seek reflexology as a treatment may receive many of the restorative benefits of other massage practices, such as stress relief and improved sleep patterns.

SPORTS MEDICINE MASSAGE

This type of massage is used to treat and prevent sports-related injuries, improve flexibility and range of motion, and enhance sports performance. Not just for professional athletes, sports medicine massage can help anyone who does regular physical activity and may need healing focused on specific muscle groups.

FINDING A GOOD MASSAGE THERAPIST

Massage does not have to be expensive to be fantastic. In fact, the best massages I've had have been outside of the traditional spa setting. It's no secret that spas mark up their services like crazy. I find the best way to find a good massage therapist is word of mouth. Ask around and you'll be surprised at how many recommendations you get for those who practice privately or will come to your home. And in today's rapid world, some brilliant minds, like the creators of the app Zeel, have figured out how to bring high-quality, moderately priced massage therapy to you. (No, I don't work for them. I just love their business.)

TALK THERAPY

I consider myself very lucky to have grown up with a psychiatrist for a dad. As I got older, I always had someone to talk to about life's problems. Sure, there were many times when I felt my parents were my biggest problem—they divorced when I was a teenager and both recoupled rather quickly—but the overall message I received from my dad was that it's OK to ask for help and share your feelings.

Throughout my adult life, I've faced challenging experiences, as we all have. My biggest were giving birth to my children and panicking about being responsible for another human being forever; choosing to be a stay-at-home mom (and realizing it wasn't right for me and returning to a career outside of the home); some physical injuries; and, certainly the most earth-shattering and paradigm-shifting of all, the end of my marriage. At all of these points in my life, I was struck with anxiety that left me panicked, sleepless, and completely worried about my children. Seeing how my dad helped others overcome their anxiety and fears around similar situations encouraged me to seek professional help early and often. His influence also removed the stigma of mental illness for me.

Simply put, therapy is the practice of speaking with a licensed and trained mental health professional to understand your past behaviors and problems. The goal? It depends on the person, but typically it is to find ways to resolve your challenges and learn healthy problem-solving techniques. Here are a number of ways to experience therapy.

- Individual: The patient and therapist are the only participants.
- Family: An entire family works with a therapist to resolve issues affecting the family unit and the individuals within the family.
- Couples: A couple works with a therapist who specializes in couples counseling to improve their romantic relationship.
- Group: Two or more people attend therapy at the same time, often discussing the same issue, such as grief or addiction. This allows participants to share their own experiences and hear others who are experiencing similar things.

There are many types of therapy and many types of therapists out there, ranging from psychiatrists—medical doctors who are able to prescribe medication and help monitor your progress—to psychologists who focus on talk therapy; licensed marriage and family therapists; social workers; and more. Some types of therapy may appeal to you more than others.

HOW TO FIND A THERAPIST

The National Alliance on Mental Illness (www.nami.org) provides very thoughtful descriptions of types of therapists and their qualifications, including an explanation of each designation's degree requirements and certifications, and which ones are able to prescribe medication.

The National Institute of Mental Health (www.nimh.nih.gov) provides thorough information on how to find a therapist in your area, as well as information on what to do if you need to speak with someone immediately. You can also ask your own doctor for recommendations for a therapist.

So much of a patient's progress in therapy depends on the relationship that's established between the client and the clinician. When meeting with a therapist for the first time, it's OK to ask a lot of questions to determine if it will be a good fit. For example, have they counseled many clients with similar issues as your own? What results have they seen? What types of therapy do they practice? What are their thoughts on using medication in conjunction with therapy to treat disorders such as anxiety and depression? How often will you need to see each other in order to see the benefits of therapy? Take note of their answers as well as the connection you feel between you and the therapist. If you're not clicking, it's totally OK to move on and find someone you're more comfortable with.

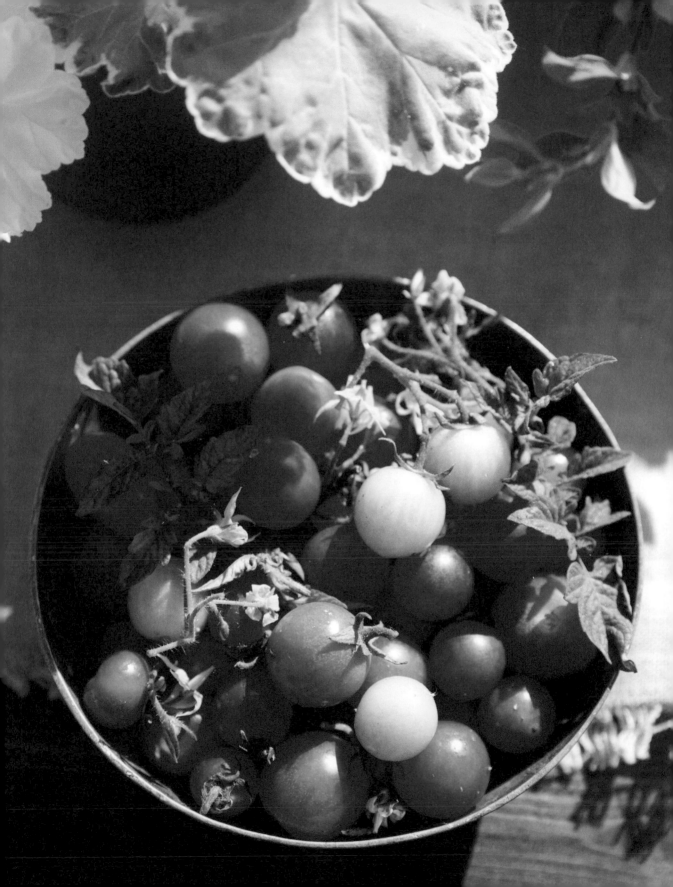

chapter

2

VEGETABLES, FRUITS, AND OTHER DELICIOUS PLANTS

After I learned about some of the best foods on the planet from Rebecca Katz (see page 52), I felt compelled to create an entire chapter focused on green foods and veggies. As she shared the health benefits of herbs, arugula, broccoli, and kale with me, I wanted to create recipes that highlighted their amazing flavors while letting their enormous health benefits shine.

In this chapter, I hope you'll find the five or six recipes that you want to make over and over again. And as you become more comfortable with vegetables taking center stage, don't be afraid to change the recipes to make them your own. Cauliflower and Romanesco are amazing substitutes for broccoli, and I'm treating arugula as the new kale. Mint can sub for basil, and tarragon can add a fragrant note to any salad or grain. So mix, match, and make these recipes work for you!

STRAWBERRY-ARUGULA SALAD

with Toasted Almonds and Mint

Vegetarian cooking hasn't always been my thing. Naturally, I tend toward steak and veggies, or chicken and veggies, or shrimp and veggies. But as I age, I can't deny that I feel better when my plate is loaded with veggies and the animal protein is a smaller part of the equation. My stomach thanks me. My waistline thanks me. My skin thanks me.

For this book, I wanted to create recipes that are loaded with veggies, protein, and as many colors of the rainbow as possible. This arugula salad packs such a punch. The quinoa provides the protein, while the strawberries are chock-full of vitamin C. And we all know by now that we need as much green in our diets as possible! To me, this is the perfect salad.

Feta can be really salty, so if you're using it, you may want to leave out the kosher salt.

PREPARATION TIME
15 minutes

SERVES
4

6 cups [240 g] baby arugula

1 cup [200 g] cooked quinoa (page 231)

1 cup [120 g] strawberries, hulled and sliced

½ cup [80 g] roasted, salted almonds, coarsely chopped

½ red onion, thinly sliced

¼ cup [8 g] chopped fresh mint leaves

Kosher salt

3 to 4 Tbsp Lemon Vinaigrette (page 223)

¼ cup [80 g] crumbled sheep's milk feta (optional)

Combine the arugula, quinoa, strawberries, almonds, onion, mint, and ½ tsp salt in a large bowl. Add 3 Tbsp of the vinaigrette and toss to coat. Taste and add the remaining 1 Tbsp vinaigrette and additional salt as desired. Sprinkle with the feta (if using) and serve.

NAPA CABBAGE SALAD

with Fennel and Roasted Almonds

Confession: I am obsessed with the food from RT Rotisserie, a casual takeout/delivery joint from the owners of Rich Table, one of my favorite restaurants in San Francisco. Although they are known for their perfectly juicy rotisserie chicken, their salads are addictive as well! I've dissected every herb, seed, lettuce, and allium that show up in their salads. This recipe is a mash-up of my two favorites. You're welcome, friends.

PREPARATION TIME
20 minutes

SERVES
4–6

---

4 cups [400 g] thinly sliced napa cabbage

1 fennel bulb, cored and thinly sliced

1 red onion, very thinly sliced

1 cup [30 g] packed fresh parsley leaves

½ cup [15 g] chopped fresh dill

¼ cup [60 ml] fresh lemon juice

2 Tbsp honey

¼ cup [60 ml] extra-virgin olive oil, plus more as needed

Kosher salt

Freshly ground pepper

1 cup [160 g] roasted, salted almonds, coarsely chopped

Combine the cabbage, fennel, onion, parsley, and dill in a large bowl.

Whisk the lemon juice and honey together in a small bowl. Slowly whisk in the oil. Season with salt and pepper. Drizzle the vinaigrette over the salad and toss to coat. Add the almonds and toss gently to combine. Taste and add additional salt, pepper, and oil as desired. Serve.

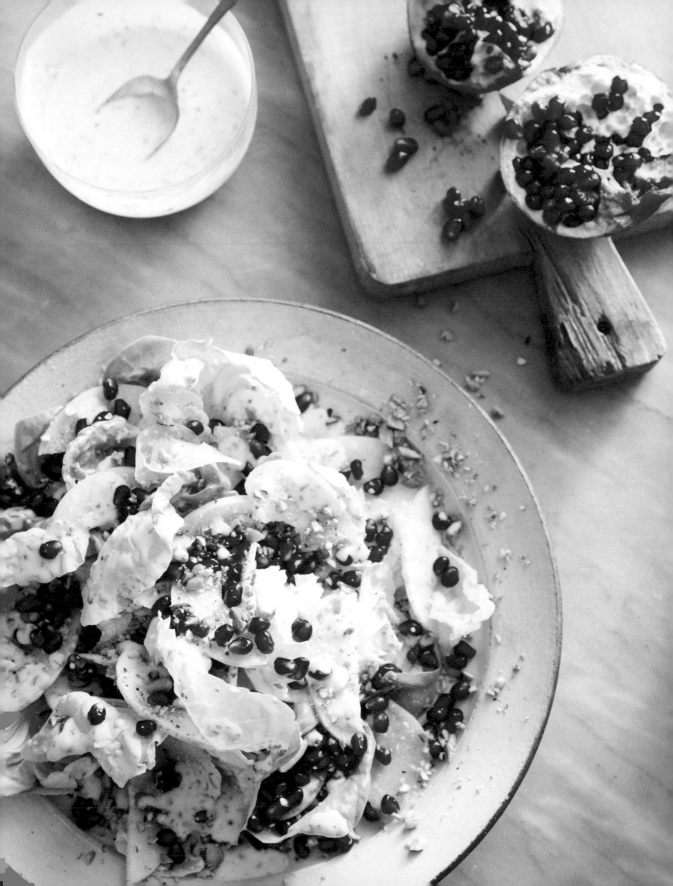

BUTTER LETTUCE SALAD

with Asian Pears, Pistachios, and Pomegranate Seeds

For me, when it comes to butter lettuce, simplicity rules. I love the texture and mild flavor so much that I don't want to hide it! So here, I add a little crunch, a little sweet, and a little savory to balance it out, then add the most divine creamy buttermilk dressing loaded with herbs. Serve this salad to people who tend to overlook them and tell me they don't come back for more!

PREPARATION TIME
20 minutes

SERVES
4

1 head butter lettuce, leaves separated	½ cup [60 g] shelled pistachios, toasted
2 small Asian pears, quartered, cored, and thinly sliced	½ cup [120 ml] Herb Buttermilk Dressing (page 222)
¾ cup [90 g] pomegranate seeds (from about 1 pomegranate)	

Combine the lettuce, Asian pears, pomegranate seeds, and pistachios in a large bowl. Drizzle with ¼ cup [60 ml] of the dressing and toss gently, adding more dressing if needed so the leaves are evenly coated yet there is no dressing left at the bottom of the bowl. Serve, passing any remaining dressing at the table.

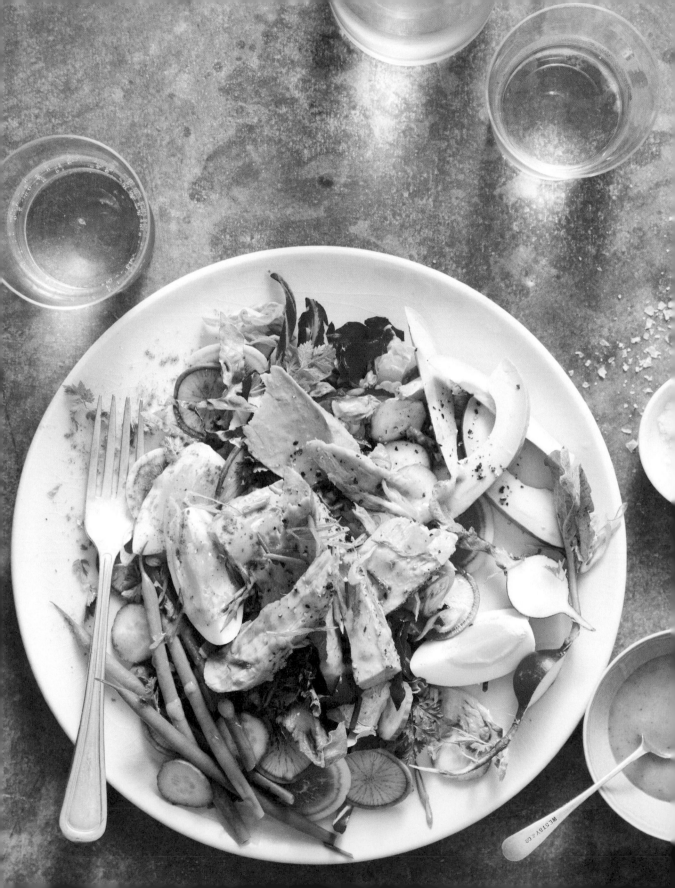

MODERN SALADE NIÇOISE

with Poached Tuna and Curry Aioli Dressing

The twist on this salade Niçoise is that the typical aioli becomes a creamy curry-infused vinaigrette, lending a depth of flavor and an anti-inflammatory punch that is often lacking.

One tip for poaching tuna: The fish needs to be completely submerged in oil to cook evenly, so use the smallest saucepan that still allows the tuna to rest flat on the bottom. Then you'll use less oil!

PREPARATION TIME
20 minutes

COOKING TIME
15 minutes

SERVES
4

POACHED TUNA

One 1 lb [455 g] ahi tuna fillet, about 1 in [2.5 cm] thick	4 strips lemon zest
Kosher salt	2 garlic cloves, peeled and smashed
Freshly ground pepper	4 cups [960 ml] olive oil, plus more as needed

CURRY AIOLI DRESSING

2 Tbsp mayonnaise	1 garlic clove, grated
2 Tbsp fresh lemon juice	¼ cup [60 ml] extra-virgin olive oil
1 Tbsp Dijon mustard	Kosher salt
2 tsp curry powder	Freshly ground pepper
2 tsp honey	1 Tbsp water, plus more as needed

CONTINUED

SALAD

2 romaine hearts, shredded	6 green onions, white and green parts only, sliced
¼ head radicchio, shredded	4 radishes, thinly sliced or quartered
3 Persian cucumbers, thinly sliced	Kosher salt
8 oz [225 g] haricots verts, blanched (optional)	Freshly ground pepper
4 hard-boiled eggs, quartered	2 Tbsp chopped fresh chives
1 avocado, sliced	

To make the tuna: Rinse the tuna and pat dry with a paper towel. Sprinkle with salt and pepper on both sides and let rest for 10 minutes.

Place the lemon zest strips and garlic in a saucepan just large enough to fit the fish. Add oil to a depth that will cover the fish, at least 1½ in [4 cm]. Heat over low heat until the oil registers 180°F [80°C]. Gently lower the fish into the oil and return the heat to 180°F [80°C]. Cook until the fish is opaque but still pink at the center, about 7 minutes. Transfer the fish to a platter or cutting board.

To make the curry aioli dressing: Whisk the mayonnaise, lemon juice, mustard, curry powder, honey, and garlic in a small bowl to combine. Slowly whisk in the oil. Season with salt and pepper. Whisk in the water to reach a pourable consistency, adding a little more if necessary. Taste and add salt and pepper as desired.

To assemble the salad: Arrange the romaine, radicchio, cucumbers, haricots verts (if using), eggs, avocado, green onions, and radishes on a platter, and season with salt and pepper. Arrange the tuna on top and sprinkle with the chives. Drizzle with the dressing and serve.

WARM SPINACH SALAD
with Beets, Apples, and Bacon Vinaigrette

Those who practice Ayurvedic medicine believe a person's health is determined not only by the foods they eat, but also by their ability to digest and metabolize those foods. So one person might digest raw foods really well, and someone else might do much better with cooked foods. With very little knowledge of true Ayurveda, I know my body simply craves and reacts better to cooked foods than to raw. So in this recipe, I riff on a traditional spinach salad with a hot bacon dressing. The hot dressing cooks the spinach enough to keep me happy while bringing out the intense flavors of all of the other vegetables.

PREPARATION TIME
15 minutes

COOKING TIME
10 minutes

SERVES
4

---

10 oz [285 g] baby spinach

2 carrots, peeled and cut into matchsticks

2 beets, roasted, peeled, and cut into ½ in [12 mm] wedges

4 green onions, white and light green parts only, thinly sliced

1 apple, cut into matchsticks

4 radishes, thinly sliced

Kosher salt

Freshly ground black pepper

6 slices center-cut bacon, diced into ½ inch [12 mm] pieces

3 Tbsp apple cider vinegar

2 Tbsp honey

1 Tbsp poppy seeds

4 oz [115 g] goat cheese, crumbled

Combine half of the spinach, the carrots, beets, green onions, apple, and radishes in a large bowl. Season with salt and pepper and set aside.

In a large skillet over medium heat, cook the bacon until crispy, 4 to 5 minutes, stirring constantly to render the fat and prevent burning. Transfer the bacon to a paper towel–lined plate until cool enough to handle. Add the bacon to the salad bowl.

Pour off all but 3 Tbsp of the bacon fat from the pan, and return the pan to low heat. Add the vinegar, honey, and poppy seeds, and whisk until the mixture begins to simmer. Add the remaining spinach to the pan and toss to coat. Cook until the spinach just begins to wilt, about 3 minutes. Add the wilted spinach and any remaining bacon fat and vinegar from the pan to the bowl with the salad. Toss to combine. Transfer to salad bowls, and divide the goat cheese evenly on top. Serve immediately.

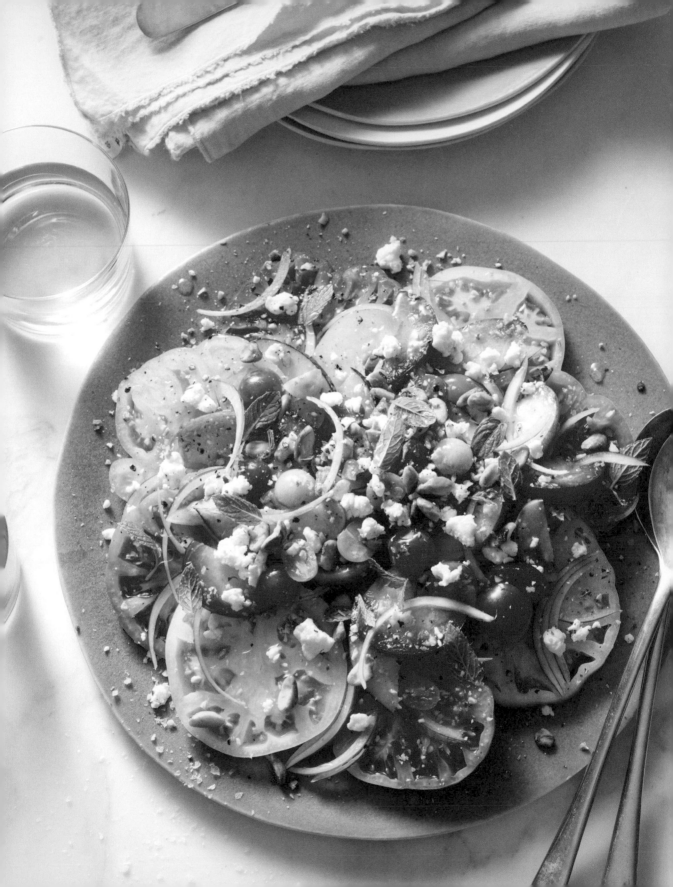

LATE SUMMER SALAD

with Heirloom Tomatoes, Stone Fruit, Goat Cheese, and Pistachios

Sharing your food with people for critique requires openness and a certain vulnerability. And after all these years of cooking for others, I still get insecure when I serve a new recipe for the first time. I shouldn't have worried with this one because I basically took everything that's wonderful about late summer and put it on a platter. My friend's teenage daughter Ella said to me, "Mandy, this is the best thing I've ever had! I didn't know I'd like peaches with goat cheese!" The secret to this recipe? Layering the ingredients so you get a taste of everything together in every bite. And not to be forgotten: I sprinkle the tomatoes evenly with the best flaked sea salt before I add anything else to the plate, so each bite bursts with that amazing tomato flavor.

If you're sensitive to nightshades like I am, you can certainly skip the tomatoes and focus on the other ingredients. Placing a sliced avocado over the top could be a nice alternative.

PREPARATION TIME
30 minutes

SERVES
6–8

6 lb [2.7 kg] heirloom tomatoes of any variety, sliced ½ in [12 mm] thick

Flaked sea salt

1 small red onion, very thinly sliced

2 lb [910 g] ripe stone fruit, such as plums, apricots, peaches, or nectarines, cut into ¼ in [6 mm] slices

½ cup [85 g] of cherry tomatoes (optional)

½ cup [60 g] lightly salted shelled pistachios

4 oz [115 g] goat cheese, crumbled

⅓ cup [10 g] loosely packed fresh mint leaves

2 to 3 Tbsp extra-virgin olive oil

Freshly ground pepper

Arrange the tomato slices in a single layer on a large platter. Sprinkle evenly with about 1 tsp flaked sea salt. Arrange the slices of red onion in an even layer over the tomatoes. Arrange the sliced stone fruit on top of the onions. Add the cherry tomatoes (if using). Sprinkle with the pistachios. Crumble the goat cheese evenly across the fruit, then tear the mint leaves and scatter over the top. Drizzle the oil over the entire salad, then season generously with salt and pepper. Serve immediately.

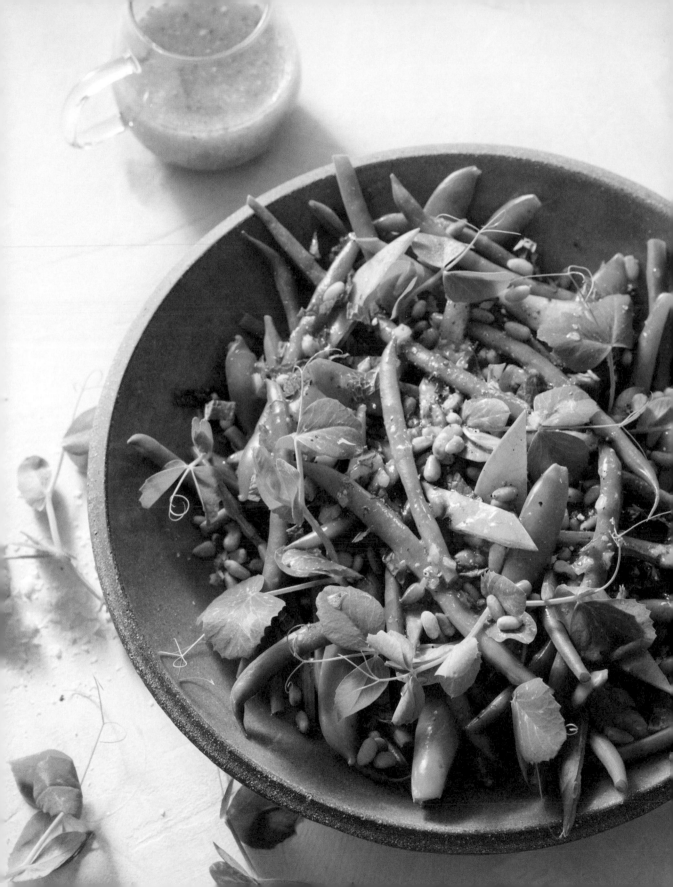

GREEN BEAN *and* SNAP PEA SALAD

with Mustard Vinaigrette

I am a huge lover of Yotam Ottolenghi's cookbooks. He can turn the simplest of vegetables into magical masterpieces. One recipe that has stuck with me is a green bean and wild rice salad with fresh tarragon and a coarse mustard vinaigrette. In my version, I use as many crunchy greens as possible to provide a contrast in textures, but you can use as many or as few as you like. Promise me you'll use coarse-grain mustard; it adds an addictive, extra pop! Thank you, Yotam, for teaching me that vegetables deserve to take center stage at the table.

PREPARATION TIME
40 minutes

COOKING TIME
10 minutes

SERVES
4–6

SALAD

Kosher salt

2 lb [910 g] green beans, trimmed

8 oz [225 g] snap peas

1 Tbsp extra-virgin olive oil

⅓ cup [55 g] pine nuts

8 oz [225 g] snow peas, trimmed and sliced on the bias

2 cups [60 g] pea shoots (optional)

½ cup [20 g] roughly chopped fresh mint or tarragon

MUSTARD VINAIGRETTE

¼ cup [60 ml] fresh lemon juice

2 Tbsp minced shallot

2 Tbsp coarse-grain mustard

1 Tbsp honey

½ cup [120 ml] extra-virgin olive oil

Kosher salt

Freshly ground black pepper

Bring a large pot of water to a boil and add 2 Tbsp salt. Prepare an ice bath in a large mixing bowl (3 parts ice to 2 parts water).

Blanch the green beans until bright green and slightly softened, about 3 minutes. Transfer to the ice bath until cooled, then transfer to a paper towel–lined plate to dry. Blanch the snap peas until bright green and slightly softened, about 2 minutes. Transfer to the ice bath, then transfer to a paper towel–lined plate.

CONTINUED

In a small skillet over medium heat, heat the oil. Add the pine nuts and a pinch of salt, and cook until fragrant and golden brown, about 3 minutes. Let cool completely.

To make the mustard vinaigrette: In a small bowl, combine the lemon juice, shallot, and mustard, and let sit for about 5 minutes. Whisk in the honey. Slowly whisk in the oil until smooth. Season with salt and pepper.

To assemble the salad: Combine the blanched green beans and snap peas and raw snow peas in a large bowl. Add the pea shoots, mint, pine nuts, and ½ cup [120 ml] of the vinaigrette. Toss to combine, adding the remaining vinaigrette as desired, and serve.

THAI RICE NOODLES
with Peppers and Asparagus

I love Thai food. With an eye toward balancing sweet, sour, salty, and umami in every bite, even the simplest Thai recipes are delicious. But my biggest health challenge when working with Thai recipes is the sodium content. I'm all for salt for seasoning my food—it truly brings out all of the flavors in a dish—but fish sauce is loaded with sodium. So here I use the smallest amount possible to still pack a ton of flavor. With its balance of fresh herbs, crunchy almonds, spicy jalapeño, and fried shallots, this recipe would make my Thai friends proud.

PREPARATION TIME
20 minutes

COOKING TIME
15 minutes

SERVES
4

FRIED SHALLOTS

1 cup [180 g] rice flour	2 shallots, thinly sliced into rings
Kosher salt	3 cups [720 ml] grapeseed oil, for frying
Freshly ground black pepper	

DRESSING

¼ cup [60 ml] fish sauce	2 garlic cloves, minced
¼ cup [60 ml] fresh lime juice	1½ tsp red pepper flakes
3 Tbsp maple syrup	Kosher salt

CONTINUED

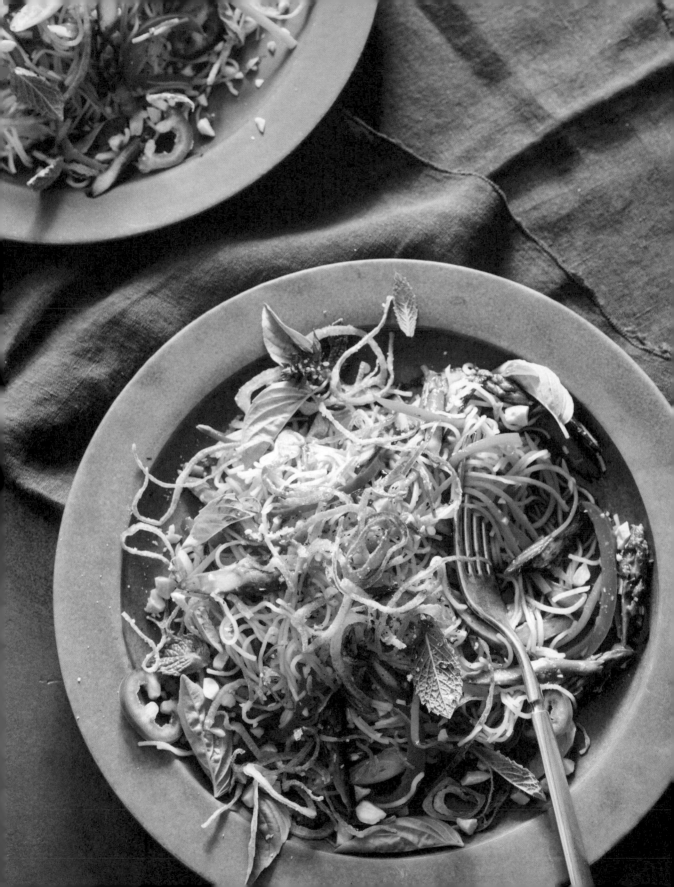

NOODLES

One 8.8 oz [250 g] box thin rice noodles	2 green onions, white and light green parts only, thinly sliced
2 Tbsp grapeseed oil	Kosher salt
1 red or yellow bell pepper, thinly sliced	Freshly ground black pepper
1 bunch asparagus, cut into 2 in [5 cm] pieces	½ cup [80 g] Marcona almonds
3 carrots, peeled and cut into matchsticks	½ cup [10 g] loosely packed mint leaves
	½ cup [10 g] loosely packed basil leaves
	1 jalapeño, thinly sliced

To make the fried shallots: In a small bowl, whisk the rice flour with a pinch each of salt and pepper. Toss the shallots in the rice flour mixture to coat. In a small saucepan, heat the grapeseed oil to 350°F [180°C]. Fry the shallots, in batches, until golden brown and crispy, 2 to 3 minutes, then transfer to a paper towel–lined plate. Season with salt and set aside.

To make the dressing: In a small bowl, whisk together the fish sauce, lime juice, maple syrup, garlic, and pepper flakes. Season with salt.

To make the noodles: Bring a large pot of water to a boil over medium heat. Add the rice noodles and cook until tender, about 7 minutes. Drain, rinse with cold water, and set aside to cool slightly. Toss with the dressing to coat.

In a skillet over high heat, warm the grapeseed oil. Cook the pepper and asparagus until charred and tender, about 3 minutes. Add to the noodles, along with the carrots and green onions. Toss to combine, and season with salt and pepper; transfer to a serving dish. Top with the almonds, mint, basil, jalapeños, and fried shallots and serve.

SEAMUS'S BUTTERNUT SQUASH SOUP

with Garlicky Panko Crumbs

Seamus Mullen is an award-winning chef from New York City. Diagnosed with rheumatoid arthritis, he nearly lost the battle when he wound up hospitalized with a 106°F [41°C] fever. From that day forward, Seamus launched an attack on his arthritis through rigorous diet changes, exercise, and the help of an incredible doctor. Six months later, Seamus began to see some relief. Today, he shows no signs of the disease.

Seamus recently came to visit and shared a soup recipe from his book *Real Food Heals*. What I loved about it was that instead of toiling over a stockpot to sauté a bunch of aromatics for soup, he simply roasted all of the ingredients on a sheet pan together, bringing out all of the flavor without the fuss. Then he popped them into a blender, added some stock, and ta-dah! the soup was finished. Here is my take on his delicious recipe.

Butternut squash is a total pain to peel and chop. Without a very sharp knife and a steady hand, you risk cutting yourself. So, if you're nervous, treat yourself and look for prepeeled, organic, diced butternut squash at the grocery store.

PREPARATION TIME
20 minutes

COOKING TIME
1 hour

SERVES
4–6

SOUP

3 lb [1.6 kg] butternut squash, peeled, seeded, and diced	Freshly ground black pepper
6 celery stalks, sliced	¼ cup [60 ml] extra-virgin olive oil
2 Tbsp fresh thyme leaves	2 tsp sherry vinegar
2 garlic cloves, peeled	½ red onion, thinly sliced
1 tsp fennel seeds	4 to 6 cups [960 ml to 1.4 L] chicken or vegetable stock
Kosher salt	1½ Tbsp fresh lemon juice

BREAD-CRUMB TOPPING

3 Tbsp extra-virgin olive oil	1 Tbsp fresh thyme leaves
1 garlic clove, minced or grated	1 Tbsp sherry vinegar
½ cup [45 g] gluten-free panko bread crumbs	Kosher salt
	Freshly ground pepper

To make the soup: Preheat the oven to 375°F [190°C]. In a large mixing bowl, toss the squash, celery, thyme, garlic, fennel seeds, 1 tsp salt, and a generous grinding of pepper with the oil and vinegar.

Divide evenly between two baking sheets, and roast for 20 minutes. Add the red onion, stir, and roast until the onion is soft and the squash can easily be pierced with a fork, about 30 minutes longer. Transfer to a wire rack and let cool.

To make the bread-crumb topping: While the vegetables are roasting, warm the oil in a large saucepan over medium heat. Add the garlic and cook just until fragrant but not burned, about 30 seconds. Add the panko and thyme, and stir to coat the crumbs. Drizzle the vinegar over the top, then season generously with salt and pepper. Cook until the crumbs are golden and crunchy, about 2 minutes. Remove from the heat.

Transfer the cooled vegetables to a blender, and add 2 cups [480 ml] of the stock. Beginning on low, blend the vegetables, turning the speed to high to puree it completely. Add 2 more cups [480 ml] of the stock and blend to combine. Depending on the consistency you prefer, add up to 2 more cups [480 ml] of stock. Add the lemon juice, and season with salt and pepper.

Ladle the soup into bowls, sprinkle with a spoonful of bread crumbs, and serve immediately.

This soup can be cooled and refrigerated for up to 3 days. If making it in advance, simply make the bread crumbs right before serving.

LENTIL MINESTRONE
with Chard, White Beans, and (Sometimes) Sausage

I always love when people make soup, but I rarely think to make it myself. Funny though—people constantly ask me for soup recipes. This minestrone is loaded with everything good for you on the planet, luckily leaving tons of flavor in its wake. That's because of the cheese rind—an inexpensive, quick way to add flavor to the simplest of soups—and loads of caramelized veggies and fresh herbs. The sausage is totally optional; it's great if you're looking to add more depth of flavor, but you certainly won't be disappointed in how hearty and filling this soup is without it. Either way, make this soup on a Sunday and look forward to eating it all week long.

PREPARATION TIME
20 minutes

COOKING TIME
1 hour

SERVES
6

1 cup [200 g] French green lentils

¼ cup [60 ml] extra-virgin olive oil

10 oz [280 g] ground mild Italian sausage (optional)

2 yellow onions, diced

2 carrots, peeled and diced

4 celery stalks, sliced

2 garlic cloves, grated

Kosher salt

Freshly ground black pepper

2 Tbsp tomato paste

2 tsp fennel seeds plus 1 Tbsp, toasted, for garnish

1 tsp dried oregano

1 tsp red pepper flakes

8 cups [2 L] chicken or vegetable stock

One 28 oz [794 g] can crushed San Marzano tomatoes

One 3 inch [7.5 cm] Parmesan cheese rind, plus grated Parmesan for garnish

One 15 oz [425 g] can white beans, drained and rinsed

1 bunch Swiss chard, stemmed and coarsely chopped

1 cup [20 g] thinly sliced fresh basil for garnish

Combine the lentils with 3 cups [720 ml] hot water in a medium bowl and let soak for 15 minutes. Drain and set aside.

In a large stockpot or Dutch oven over medium heat, warm the oil. Add the sausage (if using) and cook until well browned, about 7 minutes. Using a slotted spoon, transfer the sausage to a plate. Add the onions, carrots, and celery and cook until soft, about 8 minutes. Add the garlic, season with salt and pepper, and cook for 1 minute. Add the tomato paste, fennel seeds, oregano, and pepper flakes and continue to cook for 1 minute. Add the chicken stock, tomatoes, Parmesan rind, and drained lentils and bring to a boil. Reduce the heat to low, cover partially, and simmer until the lentils are cooked through and the stock has reduced slightly, 20 to 30 minutes. Stir in the beans and chard, increase the heat to medium, and cook until the chard softens, about 5 minutes longer. Remove the Parmesan rind from the soup and season the soup with salt and pepper. Ladle the soup into bowls. Sprinkle with the basil, toasted fennel seeds, and grated Parmesan and serve.

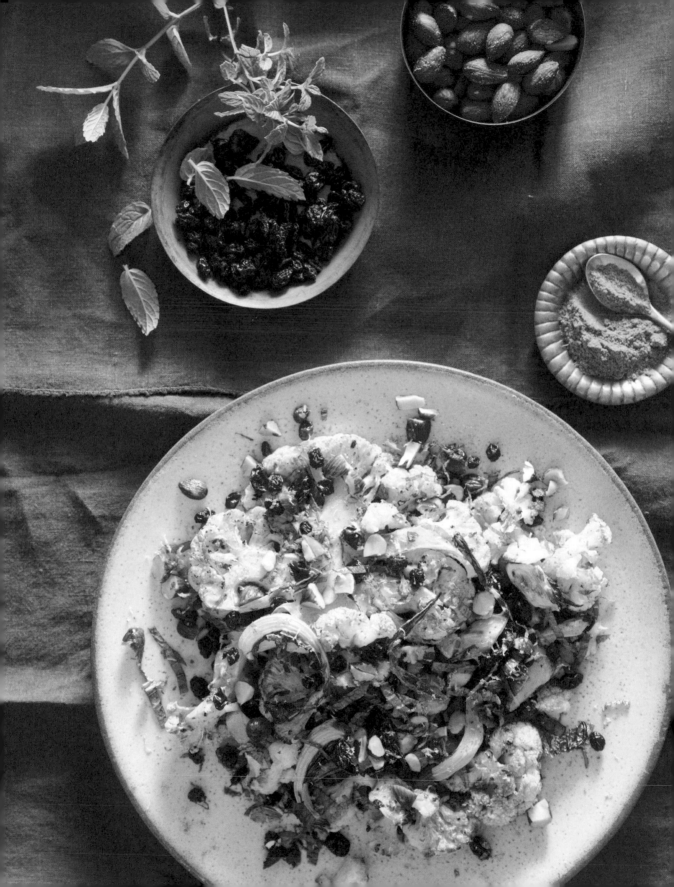

BLISTERED CURRY CAULIFLOWER

with Mint, Currants, and Toasted Almonds

When I'm left to my own devices, you'll see me roasting cauliflower for breakfast, lunch, and dinner. Proven to balance hormones, reduce cancer risk, fight inflammation, improve digestion, and even aid in weight loss, this is one underappreciated crucifer we all need in our lives! Roasted at high heat with anti-inflammatory spices and balanced with bright mint and crunchy almonds, this cauliflower is a vegetarian dream come true. Though I love chunks of cauliflower, slices cook faster and have more surface area to get crispy and caramelized. Don't forget: where there's turmeric, there should be black pepper. It increases the bio-availability of turmeric by 2000 percent!

PREPARATION TIME
15 minutes

COOKING TIME
15–20 minutes

SERVES
4

1 head cauliflower, about 1½ lb [680 g], cored and cut into ½ in [12 mm] slices	Freshly ground black pepper
2 Tbsp extra-virgin olive oil	⅓ cup [55 g] roasted, salted almonds, chopped
1 garlic clove, grated	¼ cup [45 g] currants, rehydrated and drained
1 tsp curry powder	
½ tsp ground turmeric	¼ cup [8 g] chopped fresh mint
Kosher salt	2 tsp grated lime zest

Preheat the oven to 450°F [230°C].

Combine the cauliflower, oil, garlic, curry powder, turmeric, ½ tsp salt, and ½ tsp pepper in a large bowl. Toss until the cauliflower is evenly coated. Spread the cauliflower out onto a large baking sheet, making sure not to overcrowd the cauliflower. Roast until the cauliflower is tender and golden brown, 15 to 20 minutes, flipping halfway through. Toss with the almonds, currants, mint, and lime zest. Season with salt and pepper. Serve warm or at room temperature.

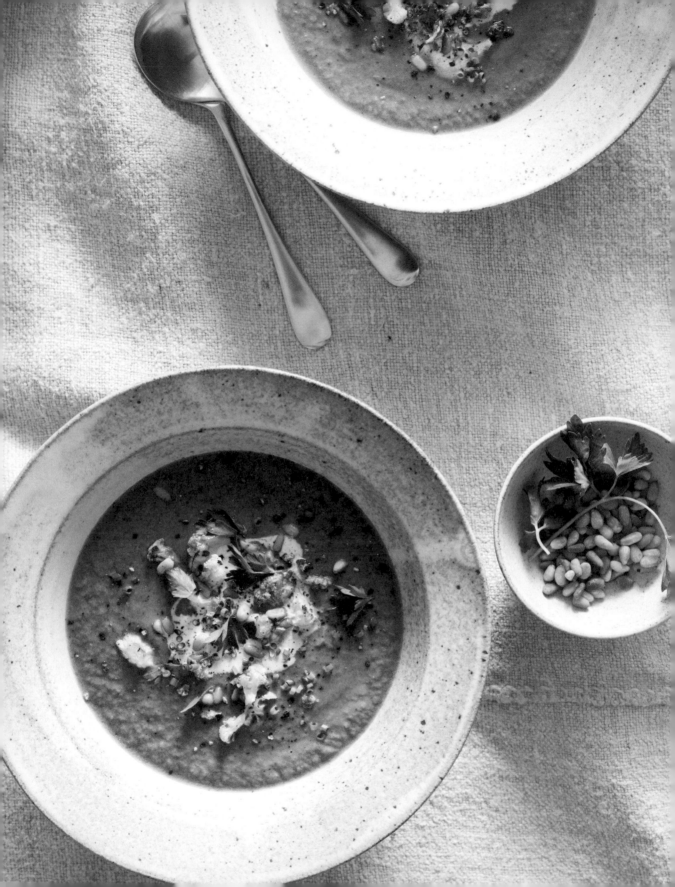

CAULIFLOWER-KALE SOUP

with Toasted Pine Nuts

I love when I can combine colors of the rainbow to create recipes that are delicious and incredibly good for you. Cauliflower and kale are both loaded with vitamin C, manganese, protein, and fiber. They also help detoxify the liver. Throw in herbs and olive oil for good measure and this soup is a total home run.

I prefer homemade chicken stock for flavor when I have it, but if you'd prefer to keep this dish vegan make sure you're using a veggie stock that has great flavor and isn't too salty (and omit the crème fraîche garnish).

For a beautiful garnish, reserve a handful of the roasted cauliflower to sprinkle on the finished soup.

PREPARATION TIME
10 minutes

COOKING TIME
45 minutes

SERVES
4

1 head cauliflower, about 1½ lb [680 g], cored and cut into 2 in [5 cm] florets

4 Tbsp [60 ml] extra-virgin olive oil

Kosher salt

Freshly ground black pepper

1 yellow onion, diced

2 garlic cloves, minced

2 bunches lacinato kale, stemmed and coarsely chopped

4 cups [960 ml] chicken stock

3 Tbsp fresh lemon juice

¼ cup [40 g] toasted pine nuts

¼ cup [60 g] crème fraîche

¼ cup [5 g] chopped fresh chives

¼ cup [5 g] fresh parsley leaves

Preheat the oven to 400°F [200°C]. In a large mixing bowl, toss the cauliflower with 2 Tbsp of the oil, and season with salt and pepper. Spread the cauliflower out onto a large baking sheet, making sure not to overcrowd the cauliflower. Roast until the cauliflower is tender and golden brown, about 20 minutes, turning the florets over halfway through. Set aside.

CONTINUED

In a large saucepan or Dutch oven over medium heat, warm the remaining 2 Tbsp olive oil. Add the onion to the pan, along with a generous pinch of salt. Cook, stirring occasionally, until translucent, 5 to 8 minutes. Add the garlic and cook until fragrant, about 1 minute more. Add the kale and continue to cook until wilted, about 5 minutes. Add the cauliflower to the pan along with the chicken stock. Bring to a simmer and cook for 10 minutes.

Remove the soup from the heat and let cool slightly. Working in batches, transfer to a blender and mix on high speed until completely smooth. Return the soup to the saucepan, and stir in the lemon juice. Season with salt and pepper. Divide between four bowls, and garnish with the pine nuts, crème fraîche, chives, and parsley. Serve.

MERRITT'S SEXY CANNELLINI BEANS

(a.k.a. Almost-Vegetarian Cassoulet)

Merritt Watts is an incomparable business colleague, friend, and wildly creative human being. Having worked with her for five years, I've come to learn that every meeting is better with her in it—she's so dang smart! So when Merritt told me she was looking for a "sexy bean recipe," I tried not to laugh out loud before promising her one. I mean, I get what she means. Beans sound so boring, being such a staple in so many diets. And let's face it; their reputation does not lead you to think you'll feel sexy after consuming them. But Merritt, I think we did it. These beans are silky, dare I say sultry, and so comforting. Lighter than a cassoulet, they're rich enough to stand on their own. A true masterpiece!

Note: Don't forget to let your beans soak overnight, then drain and rinse them. Otherwise, place them in a pot, cover them with cold water, bring it to a boil, and then turn it off immediately. Allow them to sit in the water for one hour, then drain and rinse them.

PREPARATION TIME
10 minutes

COOKING TIME
1 hour

SERVES
6–8

BEANS

½ cup [120 ml] extra-virgin olive oil, plus more for finishing	¾ cup [180 ml] white wine
1 red onion, diced	2 cups [400 g] dried cannellini beans, soaked overnight
3 carrots, peeled and diced	4 cups [480 ml] chicken stock
3 garlic cloves, minced	Kosher salt
4 anchovy fillets, mashed	2 Tbsp sherry vinegar
1 Tbsp chopped fresh thyme	Freshly ground black pepper
1 Tbsp chopped fresh rosemary	

BREAD CRUMBS

⅓ cup [80 ml] extra-virgin olive oil	1 Tbsp chopped fresh rosemary
1 cup [90 g] gluten-free panko bread crumbs	1 tsp red pepper flakes
	Kosher salt

CONTINUED

To make the beans: In a large saucepan or Dutch oven over medium-high heat, warm 2 Tbsp of the oil. Add the onion and carrots, and cook until tender, about 5 minutes. Add the garlic, anchovies, thyme, and rosemary, and cook until fragrant, about 1 minute. Add the wine and cook until reduced by half, about 3 minutes. Add the beans, chicken stock, 2 tsp salt, and the remaining 6 Tbsp [90 ml] oil. Bring to a simmer over low heat, and cook until the beans are tender, about 1 hour.

To make the bread crumbs: While the beans cook, in a large skillet over medium heat, warm the oil. Add the bread crumbs and cook, stirring frequently, until golden and crunchy, 3 to 5 minutes. Remove from the heat, and stir in the rosemary and pepper flakes. Season with salt.

Stir the vinegar into the beans, and season with salt and pepper. Top with the bread crumbs, and drizzle with a little more oil, if desired. Serve.

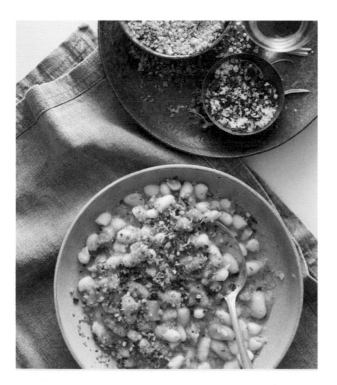

SHAVED BRUSSELS SPROUTS

with Root Vegetables and Citrus–Goat Cheese Vinaigrette

We all know Brussels sprouts are good for us—why else would so many children turn up their noses at them?—but what about the fact that they are delicious when prepared well? Roasted with apples and a little olive oil, they become sweet and candy-like. Or shaved thinly and tossed with some roasted veggies and goat cheese, as in this recipe, they sing! With every bite, you're keeping your immune system strong, and maintaining beautiful skin and teeth. Promise me you'll try this recipe once.

There are a number of ways to shave the Brussels sprouts. You can either use a knife and make very thin slices, use the thinnest blade on a food processor, or use a mandoline.

PREPARATION TIME
20 minutes

COOKING TIME
30 minutes

SERVES
6

---

1 sweet potato, peeled and cut in ½ in [12 mm] dice

2 parsnips, peeled and sliced ½ in [12 mm] thick on the bias

4 shallots, sliced ¼ in [6 mm] thick

4 Tbsp [60 ml] extra-virgin olive oil

Kosher salt

Freshly ground pepper

3 oz [85 g] goat cheese

1 tsp grated orange zest plus 5 Tbsp [75 ml] fresh orange juice

2 Tbsp champagne vinegar

2 garlic cloves, minced

1 lb [455 g] Brussels sprouts, shaved

¾ cup [90 g] pomegranate seeds

Preheat the oven to 425°F [220°F]. Combine the sweet potato, parsnips, shallots, and 2 Tbsp of the oil on a baking sheet, season with salt and pepper, and toss to coat. Spread in a single layer. Roast until the vegetables are golden and beginning to crisp, about 30 minutes. Transfer to a wire rack, and let cool to room temperature.

In a blender or food processor, mix the goat cheese, orange zest and juice, vinegar, and garlic until smooth. On low speed, slowly pour in the remaining 2 Tbsp oil, blending until combined. Season with salt and pepper.

Combine the Brussels sprouts and roasted vegetables in a large bowl. Pour the vinaigrette over the salad and toss to coat. Taste, adding more salt as desired. Sprinkle with the pomegranate seeds and toss gently. Serve.

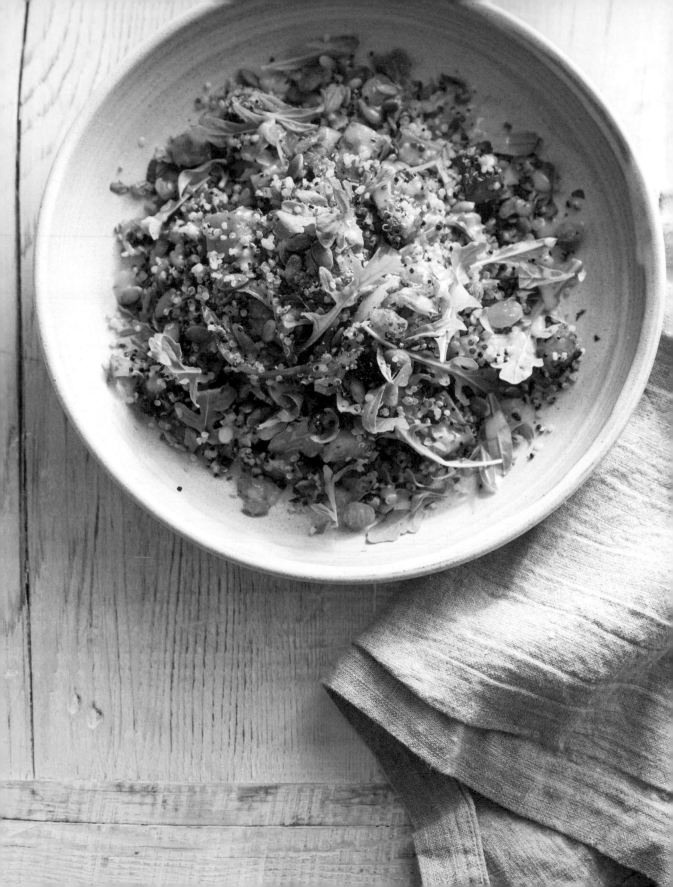

FALL QUINOA SALAD

with Butternut Squash, Toasted Pepitas, and Raisins

I've never wanted to be known for quinoa or kale, but sometimes you can't avoid your fate. My Quinoa Salad with Radishes, Currants, and Mint landed on the cover of my last book, and Gayle King—yes, THE Gayle King—was kind enough to tell me in person that she loved my Kale Salad with Quinoa and Garlic-Lemon Vinaigrette, making #gaylelovesmykale my favorite hashtag of all time!

So I'm embracing quinoa once again. Loaded with protein and the perfect swap for couscous or pastas in salads, quinoa is the perfect canvas for fall's best flavors.

PREPARATION TIME
20 minutes

COOKING TIME
1 hour

SERVES
4–6

2½ lb [1 kg] butternut squash, peeled, seeds removed, and cut into 1 in [2.5 cm] cubes

4 Tbsp [60 ml] extra-virgin olive oil

Kosher salt

Freshly ground black pepper

3 yellow onions, thinly sliced

3 cups [600 g] cooked quinoa (page 231)

3 cups [120 g] arugula

1 cup [30 g] chopped fresh parsley

¾ cup [135 g] golden raisins

½ cup [10 g] chopped fresh tarragon

⅓ cup [40 g] pepitas, toasted

½ cup Lemon Vinaigrette (page 223)

Preheat the oven to 425°F [220°F]. Place the squash on a baking sheet; add 2 Tbsp of the oil, season with salt and pepper, and toss to coat. Spread in a single layer. Roast until the squash is tender and slightly browned, about 40 minutes. Transfer to a wire rack, and let cool to room temperature.

In a large skillet over medium-low heat, warm the remaining 2 Tbsp oil. Add the onions and 1 tsp salt and cook, stirring occasionally, until caramelized, about 30 minutes. Lower the heat if the onions begin to char. Transfer to a bowl to cool completely.

In a large bowl, combine the cooked quinoa, squash, onions, arugula, parsley, raisins, tarragon, and pepitas. Add half of the vinaigrette and toss to coat, adding more if necessary. Season with salt and pepper, and serve.

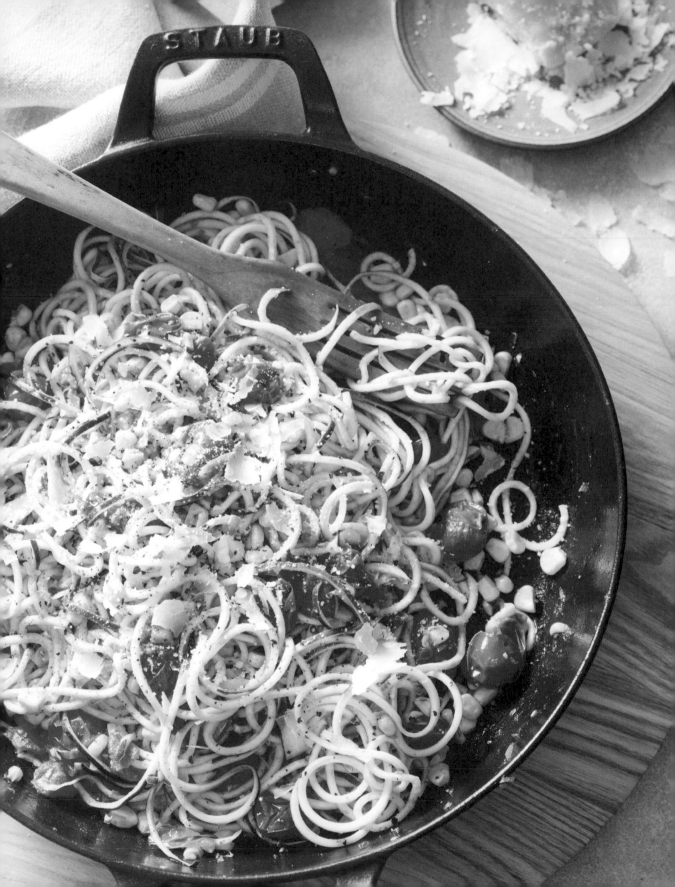

ZUCCHINI "SPAGHETTI"

with Corn and Cherry Tomatoes

Spiralizing is a craze that may be here to stay. As a gluten-free person, I love it: You can turn any vegetable on earth—from beets to zucchini—into noodles, and use them like you would pasta! It's a pretty awesome way to bring more veggies into your life without sacrificing flavor. This zucchini "pasta" is perfect for the end of summer. It uses everything that grows readily in August, and it's why these ingredients taste so good together.

PREPARATION TIME
10 minutes

COOKING TIME
7 minutes

SERVES
4

3 large zucchini

¼ cup [60 ml] extra-virgin olive oil

Kernels from 2 ears corn

2 cups [330 g] cherry tomatoes

2 garlic cloves, minced or grated

½ cup [60 g] grated Parmigiano-Reggiano, plus more for garnish

Kosher salt

Freshly ground black pepper

Use the finest blade of a spiralizer to shred the zucchini into noodles.

In a large nonstick skillet over medium-high heat, warm the oil. Add the corn kernels and tomatoes and cook, stirring occasionally, until the corn is lightly cooked and the tomatoes begin to burst, about 4 minutes. Stir in the garlic and cook until fragrant, about 1 minute. Add the zucchini and cook until just tender, about 2 minutes. Remove from the heat, and stir in the Parmigiano-Reggiano. Season with salt and pepper, sprinkle with additional Parmigiano-Reggiano, and serve immediately.

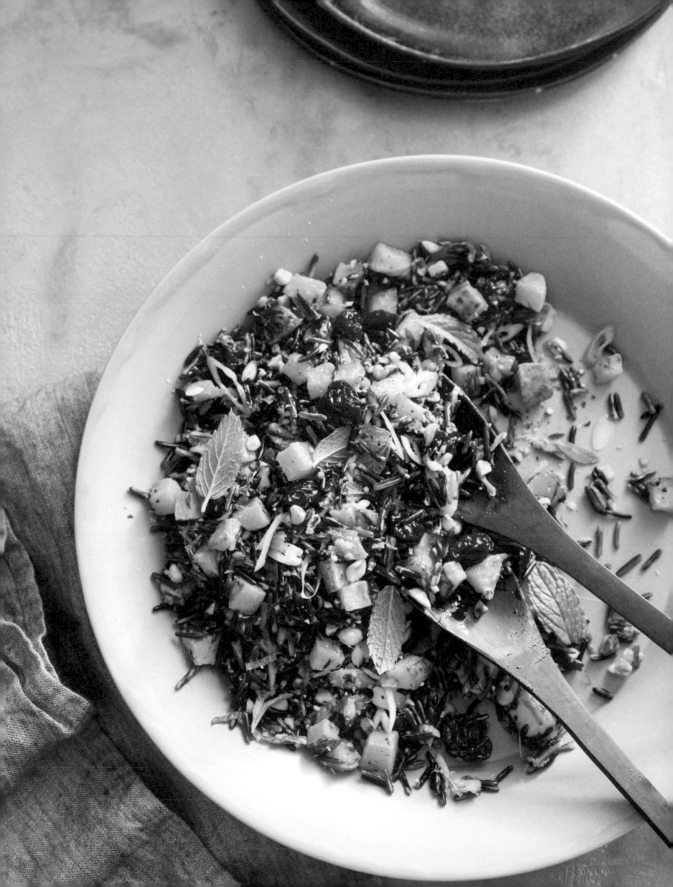

WILD RICE SALAD

with Butternut Squash, Cherries, and Mint

I've heard that when we're taking good care of ourselves, our bodies crave what they need. Well mine must need whatever is in this salad, because I find myself dreaming about it weekly! I'm also in a phase where I like to combine sweeter, richer foods like sweet potatoes and squash with a tart punch of citrus to balance things. This salad hits all of the right notes, and because it's served at room temperature, you can make it the morning of and enjoy it all day long!

PREPARATION TIME
25 minutes

COOKING TIME
4 minutes

SERVES
6–8

1½ cups [255 g] wild rice

Kosher salt

2½ lb [1 kg] butternut squash, peeled, seeded, and cut in ½ in [12 mm] dice

2 Tbsp extra-virgin olive oil

2 tsp fresh thyme leaves

Freshly ground pepper

½ cup [90 g] dried tart cherries

½ cup [60 g] shelled pistachios, toasted and chopped

½ cup [15 g] chopped fresh mint

3 green onions, white and light green parts only, thinly sliced

¼ to ½ cup [60 to 120 ml] Lime Vinaigrette (page 224)

To cook the wild rice, place in a 4 qt [3.8 L] saucepan. Add 3 cups [720 ml] of water and a generous pinch of salt. Bring to a simmer, stir, and cover. Reduce the heat to low, and cook until the rice is still a little chewy but not hard, about 40 minutes. If there is any liquid left in the pan, strain the rice. Place it on a sheet pan to cool to room temperature.

While the rice is cooking, preheat the oven to 425°F [220°C]. Combine the squash, oil, and thyme on a baking sheet, season with salt and pepper, and toss to coat. Spread in a single layer. (If necessary, use a second baking sheet.) Roast until the squash is golden and beginning to crisp, about 40 minutes. Transfer to a wire rack and let cool.

In a large bowl, combine the rice, squash, cherries, pistachios, mint, and green onions. Drizzle with ¼ cup [60 ml] of the vinaigrette and toss to combine. Season with salt, pepper, and additional vinaigrette as needed. Serve.

On Mind Body Spirit

The MEDICINE of HUMOR

with Dr. Jennifer Aaker, professor, and Naomi Bagdonas, humor expert

As the daughter of a man with one of the best senses of humor I know, I'm a true believer that laughter is the best medicine. When we laugh, even through difficult times, it can be physically and mentally transformative. Research shows that laughing even a few minutes a day can boost immunity, lower stress hormones, decrease pain, ease anxiety, and improve moods.

This made me wonder: maybe laughter is not only the best medicine—but an antiaging serum as well? I turned to two experts to find out.

The first is Jennifer Aaker, a behavioral psychologist, author, and the General Atlantic professor of marketing at Stanford Graduate School of Business. Jennifer's research has most notably focused on the psychology of time, money, and happiness—specifically, how people choose to spend their time and money, and how those choices drive lasting happiness. She's the co-author of *The Dragonfly Effect*, an award-winning book that she wrote with her husband Andy (and they still love each other!). Basically, she's a complete badass who makes me want to quit life and find a way to be accepted into Stanford Business School so I can take a few of her classes. She also weaves humor into her everyday life and is naturally funny. Her text messages often make me laugh out loud. (Example: After I came out of surgery to remove a tumor on my parathyroid gland, she asked how I was feeling. I said, "Pretty good! I'm getting a ton done and having a drink with an old friend who popped by!" She responded with, "That sounds awesome! Tumors are great for productivity!")

The second expert is Naomi Bagdonas, a corporate strategist, trained comedian, and Jennifer's partner in crime at Stanford Graduate School of Business. Together, they teach a class called "Humor: Serious Business," focused on the power and importance of humor to build more empathic, effective, and (truly) happy business leaders.

I was excited to ask Jennifer and Naomi a few questions about humor as it relates to our well-being and relationships as we age.

Amanda Haas: Is there data around how our well-being improves when we have more humor in our daily living?

Jennifer Aaker & Naomi Bagdonas: Yes, there absolutely is! Laughter releases oxytocin, which facilitates social bonding and increases trust. When people laugh together, relationships improve, and people feel more valued and trusted. And moments of laughter have lasting impact down the line as well. In one of our favorite studies, romantic couples were asked to recall times when they laughed together versus times where they shared positive moments. The couples who recalled shared laughter moments reported higher relationship satisfaction than those who simply recalled shared positive memories. So even *recalling* moments of shared laughter can make people feel better about their relationships.

And aside from improving our lives through the quality of our relationships, there are studies linking the use of humor to perceived status, confidence, and competence at work. In other words, simply landing a joke at work—as long as it's appropriate for the context—can boost your status and influence among colleagues.

AH: What happens to us if we don't have a lot of humor in our lives?

JA & NB: Death. Or at least you could make that argument. Recent research out of Stanford by Jeff Pfeffer, Stefanos Zenios, and Joel Goh (now at Harvard Business School) shows that workplace stress—fueled by long hours, job insecurity, and lack of work-life balance—contributes to at least 120,000 deaths each year and accounts for up to $190 billion in health-care costs. Therefore, mechanisms to reduce or buffer against that stress are key. Laughter makes us more physically resilient to the tensions and stressors of life. One reason is that release of oxytocin. When people laugh together at work, relationships improve, and people feel more valued and trusted, mitigating the effects of workplace stressors.

AH: What are some easy ways to incorporate more humor into your daily life? Personally I lean toward watching comedies almost nightly, hanging around funny people, and laughing at myself as much as possible.

JA & NB: Many of our students remark that they benefit from just paying more attention to humor—both when other people are funny and when they make people laugh. Humor (or even laughing) is like a muscle; it's only honed when you're working it out. (But in contrast to strengthening your biceps, humor improves when having a cocktail!)

There are techniques from comedy writing and performance that you can use to make yourself more effective at being funny, like structuring your delivery in a certain way. David Nihill has a wonderful book called *Do You Talk Funny*, full of tips and tricks to maximize small moments of humor and minimize the risks of a joke going wrong.

But we think what's more crucial in a business context is for people—and entire organizations—to engage a mind-set of levity. That is, build humor into the culture and practices of the everyday, from company meetings to new employee welcomes to otherwise mundane logistics emails. As one simple example, the two of us always take a few minutes before a class-wide logistics email goes out to make sure it has some humor in it. Even just making your text messages funny can help! I (Jennifer) have friends, like Sally Thornton and Leslie Blodgett, who make me spit out my coffee when they text me.

If you're up for a bigger time commitment, try taking an improv comedy class. Improvising unlocks a different mind-set and can make accessing your humor so much easier and more spontaneous. Most people who hear this recommendation retort that they're not funny enough for improv. We're here to assure you that (a) it's not about being funny but rather about accessing a mind-set of levity, and (b) you'll learn something directly applicable to your life or career in the process.

Humor is incredibly individualized, so discovering your own humor style and that of others is a key starting point. Then, playing or experimenting with humor, embedding it in business contexts, and amplifying it are the next layers.

AH: Can humor help us live longer?

JA & NB: That is unclear. However, a 2013 review of studies found that among elderly patients, laughter significantly alleviated the symptoms of depression. Another recent study found that firefighters who used humor as a coping strategy were somewhat protected from PTSD. But more importantly, perhaps, laughter has been shown to reduce tension and increase resilience in individuals and teams, which is particularly important in stressful times. In fact, a 1997 study that examined individuals who had recently lost a spouse found that those who reminisced about funny stories with their loved one showed lower levels of stress and increased excitement about life.

I got so much out of my conversations with Jennifer and Naomi. After speaking with them, I realized one other important thing: intelligence and humor can work so nicely together. Humor doesn't need to reduce the power of a message. In fact, it can amplify it. So often, I've held back in cracking jokes in emails or during work conversations for fear the audience won't take me seriously. But after looking at Jennifer's work and attending a few of her classes, I convinced myself I was wrong. We *need* humor to thrive, especially in a time where we work more than ever, there is more chaos in the world than ever, and we are expected to do it all. Humor truly is serious business.

My challenge to you: Find ways to laugh at life every day.

STRENGTH TRAINING *for* TOTAL BODY FITNESS

with fitness and wellness consultant Denise Henry

The truth is, as you age you lose 3 to 5 percent of your muscle mass every ten years. About 80 percent of people ages fifty and older have too little muscle and too much fat. This can lead to obesity, osteoporosis, diabetes, high blood pressure, high blood cholesterol, heart disease, stroke, arthritis, low back pain, and numerous types of cancer. Fortunately, muscle loss is reversible. And research reveals that core and strength training is an effective way to increase muscle mass at all ages.

Your core is your body's powerhouse. A strong core can reduce back pain, improve athletic performance, and help posture. In addition to rebuilding muscle, the benefits of strength training include recharging your metabolism, reducing fat, lowering resting blood pressure, increasing bone density, decreasing physical discomfort, enhancing mental health, revitalizing muscle cells, reversing physical frailty, and even combating cancer. In light of all these benefits, I had to include strength training in my book, and I turned to my friend and fitness expert Denise Henry for help.

Denise Henry and I have a long history, with roots that go all the way back to preschool. At my fifth birthday party, she gave me an Easy-Bake Oven, which sparked my love for cooking and eating. Quick-moving, athletic, and naturally hyperactive, Denise was constantly on the move. She became a very talented tennis player as a young teen, which evolved into a lifelong passion for fitness.

She's been a competitive athlete for more than thirty years and has over twenty years of teaching experience. She's a certified exercise instructor and training coach for spinning, athletic conditioning, running, core strength, and flexibility, and has studied nutrition related to sport and optimal fitness performance.

At forty-six, her body is stronger, leaner, and more flexible than it's ever been. I asked Denise for her favorite full-body exercises that help us focus on the core strength and muscle tone we need to keep our bones and bodies strong as we age.

NINE FULL-BODY STRENGTH EXERCISES

When it comes to exercising and building cardio and muscular strength, most of us would prefer to get maximum results in the shortest amount of time. Below are nine efficient exercises to get stronger faster and burn more calories in less time.

Full-body exercises will help you perform better in everyday activities as well as improve your athletic performance, making you more functionally fit. These exercises will improve muscular and cardio endurance, stamina, balance, stabilization, and mobility. Strength training can also improve your emotional and mental health.

Depending on your fitness level, you ideally want to challenge yourself to this routine at least three days a week. Repeat the exercise sequence two or three times, following the recommended number of reps per exercise.

BURPEES

Burpees are an awesome overall body strengthener and will condition you like no other exercise. With every rep, you will work your arms, chest, quads, glutes, hamstrings, and abs.

Stand up straight, then get into a squat position with your hands on the floor in front of you. Kick your feet back into a push-up position and lower your body so that your chest touches the floor. Jump and return your feet to the squat position as fast as possible and immediately jump up into the air as high as you can. Keep your core tight the entire time. Repeat ten to twenty times.

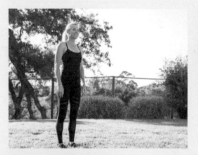
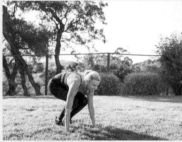
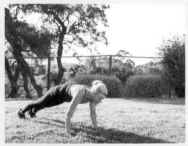
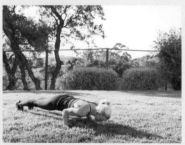
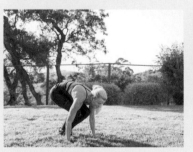
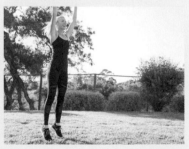

SQUATS

Done properly, squats give you a strong, powerful lower body. They will also work your core and strengthen your back and shoulders. Depending on your fitness level, you may add 5, 8, or 10 lb [2.3, 3.6, or 4.5 kg] hand weights to make squats more challenging.

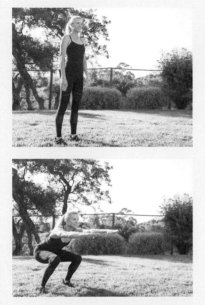

Stand with your feet hip-width apart while pulling your shoulders back and engaging your abs. Push your seat and hips back as if you're sitting in a chair. While keeping your weight on your heels, lower down until your thighs are parallel to the floor (or go lower if you can). Rise back up to the starting position, squeezing your glutes and pushing your knees outward toward your ankles as you straighten. Be sure not to let your knees come over your toes while squatting. It is extremely important to use correct form, keeping your head, shoulders, and spine neutral with your knees aligned over your ankles. Repeat ten to twenty times.

PLANKS AND PLANK VARIATIONS

Planks may be the best exercise for washboard abs! They are a basic isometric exercise that strengthens your core, lower back, shoulders, arms, and glutes.

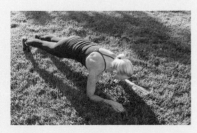

Get into a push-up position on the floor, bend your elbows 90 degrees, and rest your weight on your forearms so you are in a forearm plank position. Your elbows should be directly beneath your shoulders, and your body should form a straight line from your head to your feet with your heels, inner thighs, and glutes squeezing together. Hold the position for as long as you can, up to two minutes.

A plank can be made more difficult by removing a contact point from the floor. Try raising one foot off the ground and hold it there.

Make sure to hold your body still and keep your spine in a neutral position (no arching or rounding your back) and avoid tilting sideways. Switch legs every five to ten seconds.

A side plank targets many smaller core muscles that are often neglected. It will help sculpt your waistline and improve your posture. From plank position, press your right hand into the ground and turn your body so your weight is on the outer edge of your right foot; stack your left foot on top of your right. Press your torso up, extending your left arm straight up with your fingers pointed toward the sky. Tighten your lower ab muscles to brace your entire core and hold for thirty to sixty seconds, then return to plank position and repeat on the left side.

Alternatively, you can do a standing plank with your hands pressing into the floor and feet hip-width apart. Keep a slight bend in your elbows to ensure that your upper back, shoulders, and core take the load, rather than your neck. Standing planks strengthen your core, lower back, shoulders, arms, and glutes, with an emphasis on your shoulders and arms.

PUSH-UPS

If I had to pick my favorite exercise, it would be push-ups. Push-ups work your core, back, arms, chest, butt, and even leg muscles.

Start in a plank position with your shoulders directly over your hands (Yes . . . like the top of a *chaturanga* for you yogis). Hug your muscles into the midline of your body to tighten your abdominals, glutes, and thighs, then lower yourself down so that your chest nearly touches the floor while keeping your elbows as close to your body as possible. Keep your abs and ribs tucked in and push yourself back up into the starting position; repeat ten to twenty times. Core engagement is the key to improving your stamina with push-ups.

PUSH-UPS FOR BEGINNERS:

Find a bench or an elevated sturdy surface, about 18 to 24 in [46 to 60 cm] high so you are in a plank position on an incline with your feet on the ground. Do a full push-up from this position. Lower your chest closer to the ground as you build strength.

Alternatively, you can start in a plank position on the floor with your knees on the floor. Lower yourself down so that your chest touches the floor while keeping your elbows as close to your body as possible. Push yourself back up into the starting position and repeat.

PUSH-UPS FOR ADVANCED ATHLETES:

Start in your standing plank position and lift one leg at a time as you drop into a push-up position. You can choose to repeat the same leg or alternate legs with each repetition.

You can also try push-up jacks. To do this, keep both feet on the floor. After you lower your body toward the floor, push your upper body off the floor and clap between each push up.

STEP-UPS

Step-ups will strengthen your legs and core muscles, build endurance, and get your heart rate up all in one move. To make step-ups more challenging, add 5, 8, or 10 lb [2.3, 3.6, or 4.5 kg] hand weights, or step onto a higher surface.

Stand in front of a sturdy bench, step, or another elevated surface, pulling your shoulders back and keeping your abs tight. Set your right foot on the surface, then step up onto it, pressing through your heel, placing your left foot on the surface, and making sure your feet are flat. Step back down starting with the right leg. Repeat with your left leg. Keep your core tight as you lift and lower, and don't allow your knees to buckle in. Maintain alignment with your knee over your ankle. Repeat on each leg ten to twenty times.

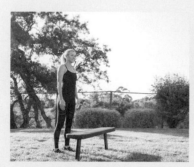 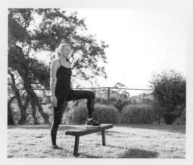 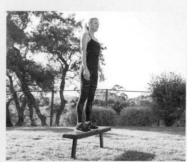

JUMP LUNGES

Jump lunges define every muscle in your legs! They will make your legs burn like crazy and get your heart rate up. This is a great challenge for your balancing skills, making it a fantastic full-body cardio and strength exercise. If you don't yet have the strength to jump from the lunge position, hold a static lunge for thirty to sixty seconds on each leg until you build up the stamina. You can make them more advanced by adding 5, 8, or 10 lb [2.3, 3.6, or 4.5 kg] hand weights or a weighted medicine ball.

Start in a lunge position with your front knee bent at a 90-degree angle and your back knee touching the floor. Jump up explosively and switch legs so that your rear leg is now in the front and your front leg is now in the rear. Repeat efficiently and quickly with proper form, keeping your knees aligned over your ankles. Repeat ten to twenty times.

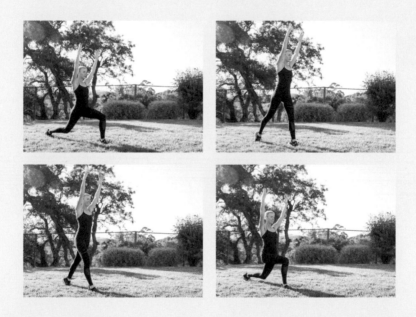

DIPS

Dips are a fantastic way to work your chest, triceps, shoulders, and abs all at once!

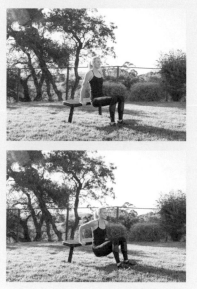

If you have access to a set of low parallel bars, stand between them and grab the bars, straighten your arms, and hoist yourself up off the ground while slightly crossing your legs. Pull your shoulders back and keep your chest up and broad, then lower yourself down so that your upper arms are parallel to the floor. Raise yourself back up to the starting position so that your arms are straight.

You can also use a bench, which is a great modification as well. Sit on a bench or sturdy surface with your feet on the floor, legs bent, and your hands behind you, elbows bent behind you (not to the sides). Raise yourself up off the bench so that your arms are straight and feet still on the ground. While keeping your shoulders back and abs tight, bend your elbows and lower your seat down toward the ground until your elbows form a 90-degree angle. Raise yourself back up and repeat ten to twenty times. To make dips more challenging, straighten your legs out in front of you.

REVERSE CRUNCHES

The reverse crunch is a basic core-strengthening exercise that also improves stability throughout the lower back, spine, and hips.

Lie on your back with your knees together, feet off the floor, and your legs bent to a 90-degree angle so your lower legs are parallel to the floor. Place your palms down by your sides on the floor for support. Tighten your abs to lift your hips off the floor as you pull your knees in toward your chest. Pause at the top of the motion, then lower back down without allowing your lower back to arch. Repeat twenty times.

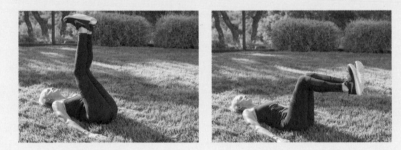

MOUNTAIN CLIMBERS

Mountain climbers are a killer exercise that fire up almost every muscle group in your body and increase your heart rate. They provide a magic combination of strength training, cardio, and core strengthening.

Start in a standing plank position with your arms and legs long, keeping your abs pulled in and your body straight. Pull your right knee into your chest and as the knee draws to the chest, pull your abs in even tighter to ensure proper form. As you push your right leg back to the starting position, quickly pull your left knee into the chest using the same form. Continue to pull the knees in right, left, right, left in a "running" motion. Stay aware of your body position. Be sure to keep a straight line in your spine and don't let your head droop. Keeping your core and body stable is essential during this exercise. Aim for ten to twenty repetitions.

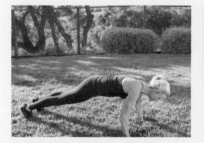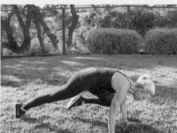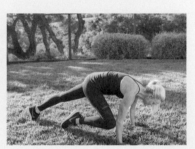

CRYOTHERAPY

When I first heard people at my gym talking about cryotherapy—also known as cold therapy—after a spin class, I thought, "They're crazy." I like to think I'm open-minded when it comes to managing my back and joint pain, but the idea of stepping into a freezer that is -180°F [-118°C] for two minutes sounded downright horrible!

But when I reinjured my lower back, I decided I'd test out the hype. I visited Tim Fitzgerald, founder of U.S. Cryotherapy in Walnut Creek, California, to see what this treatment is all about.

Cryotherapy is the therapeutic use of low temperatures, ranging from applying an ice pack to sitting in an ice bath to spending several minutes in a -180°F [-118°C] cold chamber. When applied to the whole body, cold therapy is known as WBC, or whole body cryotherapy. First explored by Dr. Yamaguchi in Japan in the late '70s and now popular in Europe, cryotherapy was designed to reduce musculoskeletal pain and inflammation. The premise is that when your skin temperature is lowered by 30 to 45°F [-1 to 7°C], your skin receptors stimulate the nervous system, causing vasoconstriction—the narrowing of the blood vessels. When you return to normal room temperature and vasodilation occurs—enlarging the blood vessels again—your body releases oxygenated blood that is nutrient-rich, helping flush out toxins and reduce inflammation. Many athletes are turning to cryotherapy for muscle recovery during intense training. I was curious about the other perceived health benefits, most notably the claims that it can reduce inflammation and help relieve muscle pain, improve energy, reduce anxiety and depression, and even promote weight loss.

There are two types of cryotherapy clinics popping up around the United States: those that use electric walk-in chambers and those that use cryosaunas. An electric walk-in chamber is like a large walk-in freezer in a restaurant—except much colder! It is cooled with a condenser with jet fans,and can fit three or four people in it comfortably. The electric walk-in chamber I was in had a very large window in the front facing out, so I could see the person operating it. (This was a huge relief as I set foot in the -220°F [-140°C] chamber for the first time!) A cryosauna is a capsule that you step into. Your head and neck are left exposed, so you can see what is happening around you. Instead of using a condenser fan to chill the space, cryosaunas use liquid nitrogen vapor.

With either method, you're asked to wear as little clothing as possible, so your skin has as much contact with the cold as possible, except for covering your most sensitive extremities.

The attendant, Tim, explained that the first session lasts for two minutes. (As your body adapts, sessions can last for up to three and a half minutes.) And luckily, he let me select a song, so the time would pass more quickly. Tim instructed me to move around slowly in the tank, rather than stand still, to help the time pass (and also to prevent windburn and shivering, yikes!). Many people do slow push-ups, squats, or stretch the areas where they're experiencing pain, in order to bring more circulation to those areas. If you move around too quickly, it can cause skin irritation because you're creating your own windchill. Slow and controlled movements enhance the experience.

I finally got up my nerve and stepped into the chamber. My first thought was, "How do I even breathe when it's this cold in here?" Then panic set in, and I thought I was going to freeze to death, but I looked out the window for reassurance from Tim. And I reminded myself that I could walk out at any time if necessary.

The cold indeed took my breath away, but after a few seconds I established my breathing and tried some slow movements the other person in the chamber suggested. Pretty soon there was a computerized voice telling me sixty seconds had passed; then ninety; and then we were in the home stretch. I'd made it!

When I stepped out of the chamber, Tim took my skin temperature. They're looking for a 30° to 45°F [-1 to 7°C] drop in the skin's temperature to reap the most benefits. (If your skin temperature doesn't drop enough, they recommend you extend your time in the chamber by fifteen to thirty seconds on your next visit.) Mine had dropped by 40° [4°C]!

After they read my temperature, for vasodilation, Tim had me hop on a bicycle and pedal slowly for five minutes (he told me that other types of light cardio would also work). The cardio helps speed up the vasodilation.

So, what did I think? After a day or so had passed, I felt less inflamed in my trouble areas. My joints felt better. It took a few more visits for me to notice a significant improvement. When I asked Tim about how many treatments you need for maximum benefits, he said it can vary greatly between people. You can use the chamber two to four times a week, but Tim reiterated to me that more than that can become too much of a good thing.

As cryotherapy becomes more popular, most medical communities agree that more research is needed to truly understand the long-term side effects and perceived health benefits of the practice. But thanks to Tim, I now see it as a viable alternative to some of the more invasive procedures I've relied on to reduce my lower back pain and joint inflammation when I have a flare-up.

SEX *and* AGING

with sex expert Pepper Schwartz

I've spent a lot of time thinking about love because it hasn't come to me in the traditional ways I expected. My marriage didn't wind up being a forever thing—it ended in 2016 after nearly twenty years. Even as those wounds are barely healing, I can already feel the new types of love forming in my life. Through my divorce, I had friends love me in a way that I didn't know was possible. Their love is starting to fill up more and more space in my life, and I feel open to all kinds of love now, including new passionate romantic love!

Since it's clear to me that we all need love in order to thrive, I started suspecting that love must be important for aging well. Then in a serendipitous twist, Dr. Pepper Schwartz walked into my life, blowing my mind with her brilliant perspective on love and sex in midlife and beyond.

Pepper is a renowned author and researcher, a very sought-after lecturer, and the star expert on the popular show *Married at First Sight*, and she continues to teach compelling, innovative classes as a professor at the University of Washington. She's devoted her life to the fields of intimacy and sexuality (and is the author of twenty-five books on the subject).

She also happens to be one of the most interesting people I've ever met. At seventy-two, she's clearly at the peak of her career. She's also a newlywed, living on a horse ranch that she built, and a passionate mother of two grown children. She travels, she rides horses, she's always game for a night out, and she's an amazing conversationalist. I like to say that Pepper talks about sex the way I talk about cooking—as a natural part of daily life that's so important for health and happiness.

One of the first questions I asked her was, "What do we need from a romantic relationship at thirty versus at sixty?" Pepper's response stopped me in my tracks. She said, "Well, we're not all the same age at the same age."

I instantly understood what she meant. Take Pepper, for example. Her version of seventy-two is many women's version of fifty-five! We're all different. So instead of focusing on sex and love at specific ages, we talked about how love and sex benefit us at any age.

Can you conjure up that feeling you got the first time you had a romantic crush? The heart-pounding, palms-sweating, mind-racing euphoria you felt? The all-consuming mind-body connection? It's powerful.

Yet so many of us write off falling in love and having great sex as we age, thinking it's something only meant for the younger folks. But that's absolutely not the case—and Pepper's here to back me up.

Amanda Haas: **I've been thinking about this a lot since my divorce—how do relationships affect our health?**

Pepper Schwartz: Love, when it goes well, turns on all our lights, energizes our entire endocrine system, and gives us the will to power through the tough moments that are inevitably part of life. Happy, loving moments release endorphins that make us feel elated, the proverbial "walking on air" feeling. When we feel loved, we feel strong, worthy, and capable. Conversely, toxic relationships, rocky marriages, and even negative family or friend encounters can depress us and create anxiety, self-doubt, and anger. These emotions raise your cortisol levels, indicating that the body is experiencing unhealthy stress. This is just one example of how our body and emotions are intrinsically linked. Think, for instance, about how dangerous depression is and how it can make someone ineffective at work, struggle to communicate with loved ones, and even lead to self-destructive behaviors. Looking at it holistically, love is a gift of health as well as happiness, while toxic relationships or isolation affect us in the opposite way and can sadly have the power to wreck our overall well-being.

Friendship has many of the same elements of a love affair, except that it doesn't include sexual attraction—for most people anyhow. The happiness of a strong friendship arises from feeling like you see the world in the same way, have similar values, truly like and admire each other, and prefer each other's company over most people's. Instead of a charge from sexual attraction, there's warmth that comes from knowing your friend has your back and wants you to succeed and be happy. Good friends are willing to celebrate your highs and help you get past your lows. There is a lot of data to support that friendship is important for our health, including a comprehensive study done at Brigham Young Medical School. The study says the strength of intimate social networks is more responsible for mental and physical well-being than whether or not someone smokes, has heart problems, or has to contend with serious disease like diabetes. We are animals that need, not just want, the company of others of our kind.

AH: **I've heard people say this, but can sex really help slow the aging process?**

PS: I love this question. My answer is yes, yes, and yes again! The production of hormones that happens when we experience physical touch is critical to our sense of youth. These hormones actually make us more physically active and emotionally buoyant. Most dramatically, when we have an orgasm, we produce greater quantities of oxytocin, the aptly named "bliss hormone," which makes us feel connected, content, and at peace.

Dopamine, the hormone associated with passionate love, makes us feel more alive—physically and emotionally turned on. Dopamine is increased with the intense longing for another, including focused (sometimes even obsessional) thinking of a loved one or desired person. Sex is part of yearning for that deeper, incredibly special connection—that "walking on air" feeling that's associated with youth. Arousal and desire are very powerful, no matter how old we are. Intercourse and orgasm also keep our bodies flexible and our circulation flowing, and they produce hormones that protect our mood and activity.

The best part? You don't need a partner in order to reap the benefits of sex. Many of the benefits of partnered sex are available through masturbation. In fact, there was a wonderful 2004 article in the *Journal of the American Medical Association* that looked at sex and prostate cancer and found that twenty-one or more "emissions" a month would help men lower their risk of prostate cancer. Those emissions were "by any means necessary." The point is, if you have an orgasm during masturbation, it will give you some of the same benefits as when it happens during intercourse or from being touched to orgasm by a partner. Of course being connected to someone else has additional benefits that come from being touched, stroked, and emotionally connected, but masturbation will keep all those body parts oiled during times when you don't have or want a partner.

On the flip side, if we stop experiencing orgasms, we can be affected physically as we age. Think about it—what would happen to your left arm if you decided not to use it for a few years? It would lose muscle tone and strength and need some very serious rehabilitative exercises in order to get back full mobility and function. The same is true with sex and our sexual organs. Without intromission for some time, the vaginal tissue, for example, can become brittle and painful. And men experience their own issues if they don't orgasm regularly. According to the *Journal of the American Medical Association*, they can be prone to more prostate infections, and there might be psychological complications from not having regular erections with a partner. A loss of confidence can easily increase the chance of erectile dysfunction.

The takeaway here is that there are many benefits to being sexual, many costs to stopping having a sexual life, and that it is worth the effort to keep your body in good sexual health as you age. Masturbation, despite the stigma attached to it, can be a great way to keep your sexual response alive and well.

AH: How does our physical health relate to our sexual ability?

PS: In order to have great sex—at any age—being in great health really matters. Athletes keep in top condition, and their top physical condition allows them to do a lot of things they may take for granted, like not running out of breath running up a flight of stairs, being able to be in a sexual position without getting tired, and being extremely active during sex because they're physically fit.

This means that going to the gym regularly isn't only about great abs or defined arms. Staying fit also makes us feel healthy, strong, and more confident about showing our body or trying new positions. Core strength and decent balance come in handy in the bedroom! Pilates in particular is great for having more intense orgasms because it strengthens the pelvic muscles, which helps create the muscle tension many of us need in order to have intense orgasms.

Mental health is important, too. Studies show that women who like sex and are generally confident are more likely to use more sexual positions. Feeling sexy, desired, and desiring boosts our self-esteem. Plus, after a climax our mood improves and we feel more rested and blissful.

We are a complete package—our mental and physical shape affect every part of our lives, and certainly our sexual relationships and personal sexual satisfaction.

AH: **What about the myth that women lose their libido after menopause?**

PS: I am not going to brag, but . . . I'm here to tell you that you can have amazing sex into your seventies and eighties! Of course you can, but let's be realistic . . .

The loss of libido for both men and women has three likely causes— and they're all fixable. If you're already in a couple, barring any physical cause, lower libido is usually due to boredom, anger, or self-loathing. These all require attention to what is (or is not) happening in the relationship, and in your own head. Time spent in therapy, couples or individual, can address these issues effectively. If you're single, then sexual reawakening has to begin with thinking about why you are alone and then putting in the effort to find a partner. I believe that sexual interest can shut down in the same way our appetite for food decreases when we've gotten into a habit of eating very little. The truth is that we can rebuild all kinds of appetites!

There's also substantial data indicating that women who loved sex before menopause are very likely to love it afterwards, whereas women who were ambivalent or negative about sex before menopause are significantly more likely to find sex after menopause more difficult or less interesting. This is not to say "it's all in their head"—it isn't—but it's also true that our sex lives aren't doomed by aging, and our attitude matters.

Perhaps more challenging to fix are the physical causes. For instance, your libido may be suppressed by powerful medications including some antidepressants, heart or diabetes medications, or other strong and necessary drugs. But even if this is the case, a doctor who specializes in sexual medicine should be able to offer some help. Post-menopausal women can have a tougher time having an orgasm due to inhibited blood flow to the vulva or a more difficult time with intercourse because of reduced lubrication or more fragile vaginal tissues—but there are solutions to these issues and again, your doctor can help point you in the right direction.

For men in their seventies and up, blood flow to the penis is typically diminished. They may also have increasing erectile problems because of diabetes, being overweight, or a vasoconstriction causing blood flow difficulties due to long years of drinking or smoking. They'll likely need to be willing to take an erectile dysfunction drug and talk to their doctor about sexual health.

The supporting factor for libido later in life, found in a 2013 AARP study and also studies coming out of Indiana University, is having good overall health—and for women, a steady partner. The bottom line is that if you want to reclaim (or never lose) your libido, it's absolutely possible.

The BENEFITS of ACUPUNCTURE

Among Eastern medicine practices that have made their way to the United States, acupuncture has become one of the most widely accepted forms of alternative treatment. But we've all seen pictures or scenes in movies where the person receiving acupuncture is covered like a porcupine with needles. It can look terrifying! So why has it gone mainstream? It works!

I've had acupuncture more than three dozen times for all kinds of health challenges. I quickly got over the idea of it being scary, because I found relief from back pain, sleep disruption, and stomach pain after acupuncture. Plus, if you're working with a good practitioner, the needles don't hurt!

WHAT IS ACUPUNCTURE?

Acupuncture has been a fundamental part of the Chinese healing system for over 2,500 years. The general theory of how acupuncture works is similar to acupressure. The theory is that there are patterns of energy—qi—flowing through our bodies that are essential for health. Disruptions in energy flow cause pain, illness, or disease. By stimulating specific anatomical points with needles—often placing the needles along key meridian points that correspond to blockages in the body—your body naturally corrects the imbalances of energy flow.

There are a variety of approaches to acupuncture in America that incorporate medical traditions from China, Japan, Korea, and other countries. The most frequent execution of acupuncture employs penetration of the skin by thin, solid, metallic needles, which are manipulated manually or by electrical stimulation. The needles are only inserted into a very thin layer of skin.

WHAT AILMENTS CAN ACUPUNCTURE TREAT?

The World Health Organization credits acupuncture with treating a variety of health issues, including nausea, stroke, hypertension, chronic muscle and joint pain, stress, insomnia, addiction, and depression, with minimal side effects. (That's a pretty positive endorsement to me!)

HOW DO YOU FIND A GOOD ACUPUNCTURIST?

I've found three great acupuncturists through friends. As with a therapist or massage therapist, it's a very personal relationship. The person you are working with will be placing needles all over your body. A level of trust needs to be established very quickly. The American Academy of Medical Acupuncture (www.medicalacupuncture.org) has a list of references nationwide. Don't be afraid to meet with an acupuncturist for an initial visit before deciding whether you'd like treatment from them.

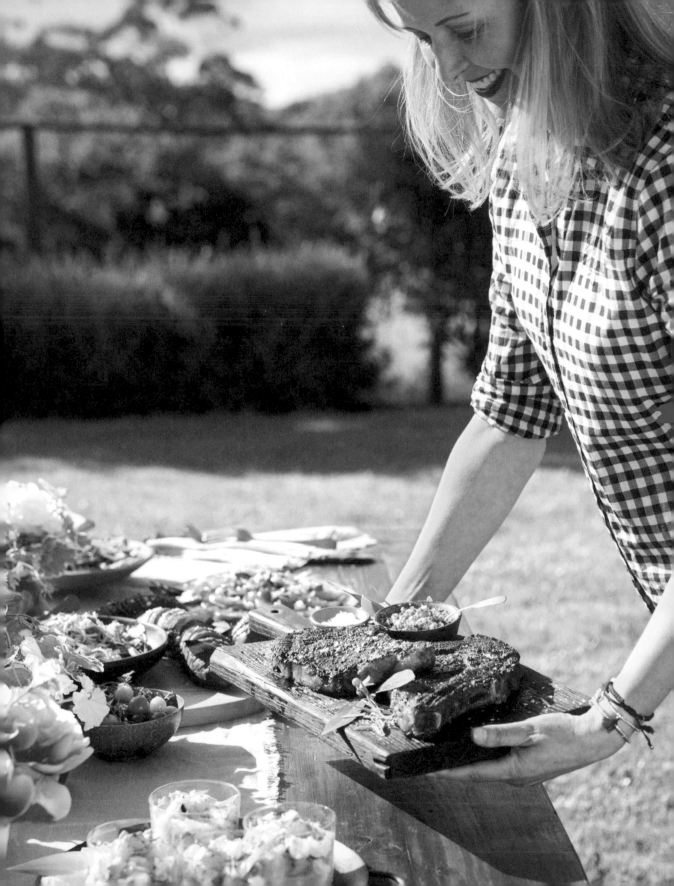

chapter

3

LAND AND SEA

I was raised eating lots of boneless, skinless chicken, a little bit of fish that came out of a Styrofoam pack from the "butcher," and even less red meat because my mom believed that carbohydrates, margarine, and low-fat ingredients were the way to go. (They were certainly the trend.) We've come a long way in our beliefs around food since the '70s! Most medical researchers now preach the importance of a diet rich in vegetables, fruits, and real ingredients. In addition, time, medical research, and common sense have concluded that we should be consuming less animal protein, especially when animals are raised in harmful environments and fed harmful ingredients, forever altering the composition of the meat. That means we're consuming all of those ingredients as well, which can wreak havoc on our bodies. (We truly are what we eat.) Raising animals for consumption is also hard on the planet, producing more greenhouse gases and using an unbelievable amount of water compared to fruits and vegetables. Garden Day Network (www.earthday.org) shares in their encouragement of "Meatless Monday" that if we eat one less burger a week, it is the equivalent of taking a car off the road for 320 miles [515 kilometers]. Isn't that incredible?

But what about consuming animal protein that has been raised responsibly and ethically, and is better for us? I like to use grass-fed beef as an example. The diet of the cattle can alter the nutrients and fats you get from eating the different types of beef. When cattle are fed grass and other foraged foods instead of corn and other grains, the beef may have heart-health benefits, including more omega-3 fatty acids, linoleic acid (a fat believed to reduce heart disease), and antioxidants such as vitamin E. Eating a piece of grass-fed skirt steak versus a grain-fed one can have a completely different effect on your body.

Eating animal protein is a personal choice. I eat it because my body feels best when I'm eating lots of veggies and small amounts of animal protein. What's different for me is that I've drastically altered how I source it. Now, I look for grass-fed organic beef, fish that comes from clean rivers and oceans, and poultry and eggs that are raised humanely and organically. And lucky for us, responsibly raised meat is becoming easier to find, thanks to Anya Fernald of Belcampo Meat, Snake River Farms, the amazing online purveyor Butcher Box, and more. When I eat this way, I simply feel better, and it shows! The food tastes better and is better for us. If you'd prefer not to eat meat, many of these recipes are delicious with vegetarian substitutes, like mushrooms, tofu, or beans.

CHICKEN IN LETTUCE CUPS

with Crispy Pine Nuts and Lime

This is my clean version of minced squab in lettuce cups, a traditional dish from Hong Kong. Instead of squab, this Americanized version uses minced chicken thighs, which work just as well. To create crunchy lettuce leaves that are the perfect vessel for the warm chicken, soak the leaves in very cold water or chill them until you're ready to serve. The crunch of the lettuce against the warm meat and veggies is irresistible. Ground chicken thighs have the fat needed to give this dish some real flavor. You can substitute ground pork for some (or all) of the chicken thigh meat, but skip the chicken breast for sure!

PREPARATION TIME	COOKING TIME	SERVES
10 minutes	10 minutes	4

2 Tbsp coconut aminos

1 Tbsp fresh lime juice, plus more as needed, and lime wedges for serving

2 tsp fish sauce, plus more as needed

3 Tbsp toasted sesame oil

1 large celery stalk, finely diced

2 Tbsp pine nuts

2 green onions, white and light green parts only, sliced, plus more for garnish

5 oz [140 g] shiitake mushrooms, stemmed and sliced

2 garlic cloves, minced

1 tsp grated fresh ginger

1 lb [455 g] ground chicken thigh meat

Kosher salt

¼ cup [10 g] thinly sliced fresh basil

12 inner leaves iceberg or butter lettuce, trimmed and chilled

Black sesame seeds for garnish

In a small bowl, whisk together the coconut aminos, lime juice, and fish sauce. In a large wok or nonstick skillet over medium-high heat, heat 2 Tbsp of the sesame oil. Add the celery and pine nuts and cook, stirring frequently, for 2 minutes, or until the pine nuts are just starting to brown. Add the green onions and mushrooms, and cook until the mushrooms start to soften, 2 to 3 minutes longer. Add the garlic and ginger, and cook until fragrant, about 1 minute. Transfer the vegetables to a bowl, and return the pan to the stove.

CONTINUED

When the pan is very hot, add the remaining 1 Tbsp sesame oil. Add the chicken and a generous pinch of salt. Stir constantly, breaking up the meat with your spatula, until it's barely cooked through, 3 to 5 minutes. Turn off the heat, return the vegetable mixture to the pan, and pour in the coconut aminos mixture. Stir to coat. Taste, adding salt, fish sauce, or lime juice as needed. Stir in the chopped basil.

Place a generous scoop of the chicken mixture inside each lettuce cup. Sprinkle with sliced green onions and sesame seeds. Serve with lime wedges on the side.

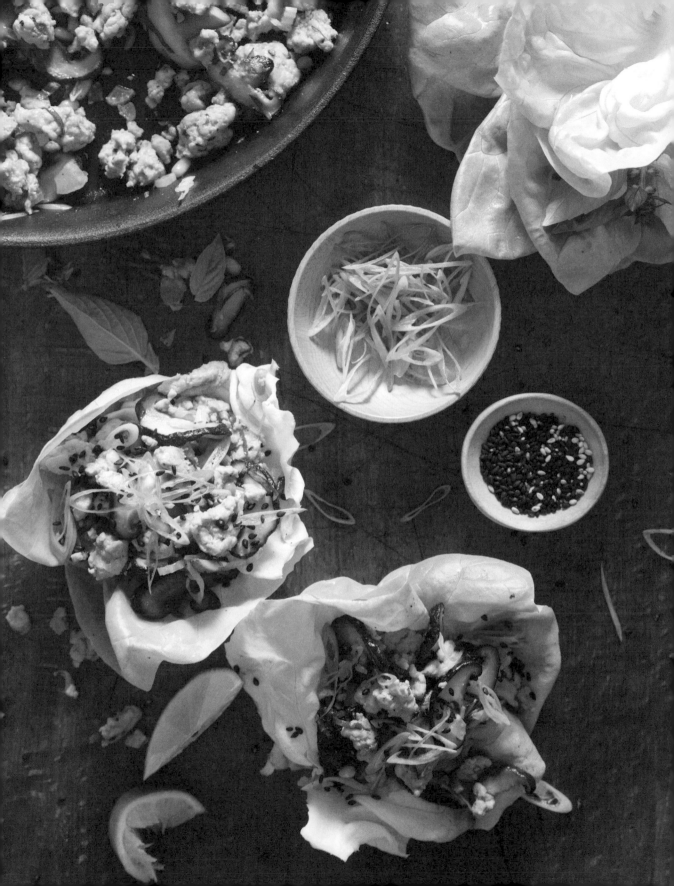

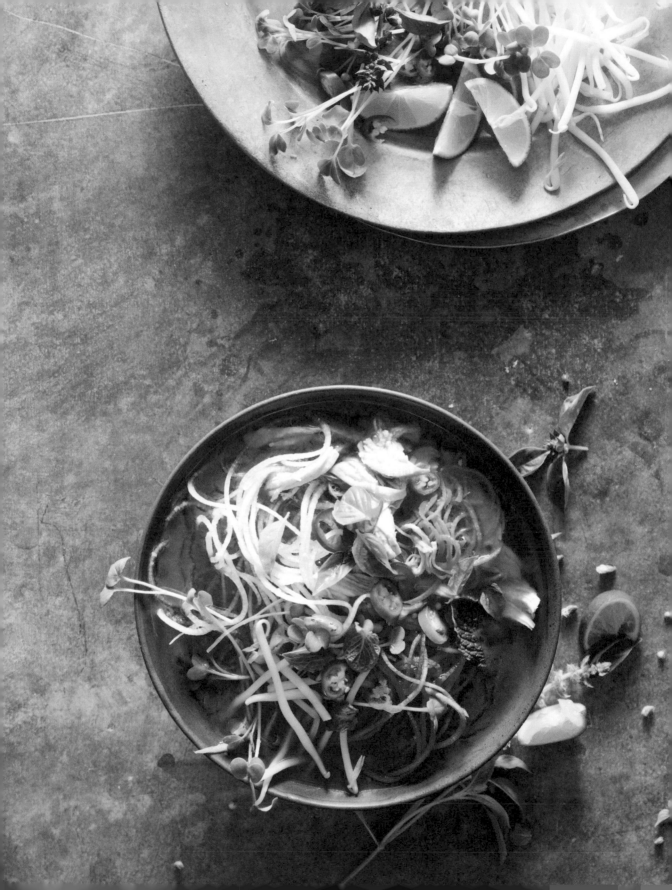

CHICKEN PHO

with Daikon "Noodles"

Pho is a cure-all soup, the Vietnamese equivalent of chicken and dumplings or chicken noodle soup. For me, it is the perfect chicken soup. Charles Phan, chef and owner of the famed Slanted Door here in San Francisco, makes the best pho I've ever had. His secrets? Coaxing every last bit of flavor out of his chicken for stock, and roasting the ginger and onions in the oven first for extra flavor.

When I've got the time, I love to do it his way, and take hours to roast the veggies and allow the stock to really take shape. But in this new version, I've done two things: I've sped it up for weeknight/easy weekend cooking, and I've replaced the traditional rice noodle with spiralized daikon radish, which is rich in vitamins and minerals and is a natural decongestant.

Coupled with the benefits of citrus and garlic, the daikon makes this soup restorative as well as a wonderful age-defying remedy.

If you prefer, watermelon radish and carrots can be used instead of, or in addition to, the daikon for a beautiful effect.

PREPARATION TIME
20 minutes

COOKING TIME
1 hour

SERVES
4

2 onions, unpeeled, halved

One 2 in [5 cm] piece ginger, thinly sliced into coins

3 Tbsp extra-virgin olive oil

4 garlic cloves, minced

8 cups [2 L] chicken stock (preferably homemade, page 230)

1 Tbsp fish sauce, plus more as needed

2 bone-in, skin-on chicken breasts (18 oz [510 g] total)

1 lb [455 g] daikon radish, peeled and ends trimmed

2 Tbsp fresh lime juice, plus more as needed

1 tsp tamari, plus more as needed

Sliced jalapeños, bean sprouts, whole basil and mint leaves, and lime wedges for garnish

CONTINUED

Preheat the oven to 400°F [200°C]. Place the onion halves and ginger coins on a parchment-lined baking sheet. Drizzle with 2 Tbsp of the oil and toss to coat. Roast until the onions are golden brown, about 30 minutes.

In a large saucepan or Dutch oven over medium heat, warm the remaining 1 Tbsp oil. Add the garlic along with the roasted onions and ginger. Cook until fragrant, about 1 minute. Add the chicken stock and fish sauce, and stir. Add the chicken to the pot. Bring the mixture to a boil, then reduce to a simmer. Cook until the chicken is cooked through, 20 to 25 minutes.

While the chicken simmers, use the finest blade of a spiralizer to shred the daikon into noodles, cutting them into about 12 in [30 cm] lengths.

Using tongs, transfer the chicken breasts to a plate. Let cool slightly, then carefully remove the skin from the chicken and discard. Remove the meat from the bones, and use two forks to shred it into bite-size pieces.

Strain the broth into a clean pot, and discard the onion and ginger. Return the chicken meat to the broth, along with the lime juice and tamari. Taste and season with additional fish sauce, lime juice, and tamari as desired.

Divide the daikon evenly among serving bowls. Ladle the soup into the bowls. Top with jalapeños, bean sprouts, basil, mint, and lime wedges. Serve.

ROASTED MOROCCAN CHICKEN

with Cauliflower "Couscous"

I am a complete couscous addict. To me, the word signifies the entire Moroccan meal of spice-rubbed and braised chicken, served with its delicious juices over a bed of couscous, the tiny wheat-based "pasta" that is typically steamed in Morocco. Well, now I am gluten-free and couscous is no longer a part of my life, but there's no need to fret. Cauliflower "rice" is a delicious alternative and works perfectly to soak up the juices from this flavorful chicken. Instead of cutting up a whole chicken and browning the pieces individually, I prefer to rub an entire chicken with the spice blend and then roast it whole for ease and flavor. While it roasts, you can make the cauliflower and herb sauce, and voilà! You've got the perfect meal for entertaining or for a family dinner.

PREPARATION TIME
45 minutes
(plus 2 hours to marinate)

COOKING TIME
1¼ hours

SERVES
4–6

SPICE BLEND

4 tsp ground cinnamon	2 tsp ground cumin
2 tsp ground coriander	1 tsp ground cardamom
2 tsp ground turmeric	

CHICKEN

4 Tbsp [60 ml] extra-virgin olive oil	5 carrots, peeled and sliced into 2 in [5 cm] chunks
2 garlic cloves, grated	4 parsnips, peeled and sliced into 2 in [5 cm] chunks
Kosher salt	
Freshly ground pepper	2 red onions, quartered
One 4 lb [1.8 kg] chicken, rinsed and thoroughly dried inside and out	2 cups red seedless grapes on the stem, cut into small bunches

CONTINUED

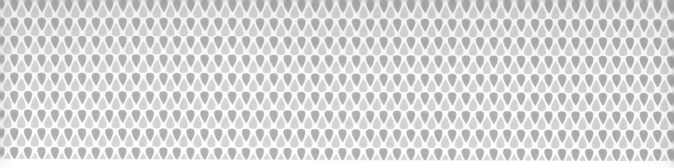

CHERMOULA

½ cup [120 ml] extra-virgin olive oil	1½ Tbsp fresh lemon juice, plus more as needed
½ cup [15 g] coarsely chopped fresh parsley	1 garlic clove, grated
½ cup [15 g] coarsely chopped fresh mint	Kosher salt
1 Tbsp minced preserved lemon	Freshly ground black pepper

CAULIFLOWER COUSCOUS

1 head cauliflower, about 1½ lb [680 g], cut in half	½ cup [60 g] unsalted shelled pistachios, toasted
2 Tbsp extra-virgin olive oil	½ cup [90 g] dried cherries
1½ Tbsp fresh lemon juice	Kosher salt
	Freshly ground black pepper

To make the spice blend: Combine the cinnamon, coriander, turmeric, cumin, and cardamom in a small bowl.

To make the chicken: In a large bowl, combine 2 Tbsp of the oil, the garlic, 1 Tbsp salt, 1 tsp pepper, and 2 Tbsp of the spice blend. Set the chicken in the bowl, and rub it all over with the spice mixture. Cover and refrigerate for at least 2 hours, or up to overnight.

One hour before cooking, remove the chicken from the refrigerator and allow it to come to room temperature. Preheat the oven to 400°F [200°C].

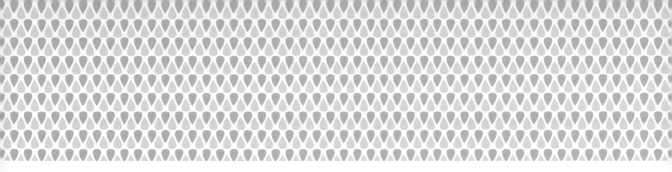

Place a roasting rack in a large roasting pan. In a large bowl, combine the carrots, parsnips, red onions, remaining 2 Tbsp oil, 1 tsp salt, and 1 Tbsp of the spice blend and season with pepper. Toss to combine, then pour the vegetables into the bottom of the roasting pan around the rack. Place the chicken breast-side up on the rack. Roast for 30 minutes, then remove the pan from the oven. Spoon some of the juices from the chicken over the top and place it back in the oven. Roast until the breast meat registers 165°F [74°C] and the thigh meat registers 175°F [80°C], or until the juices run clear when pierced with a fork, 30 to 40 minutes, adding the grapes for the last 10 minutes. Transfer the chicken to a cutting board, and tent it with aluminum foil. Let rest for 15 minutes before carving.

While the chicken is roasting, make the chermoula: Combine the oil, parsley, mint, preserved lemon, lemon juice, and garlic in a small bowl. Taste and season with salt, pepper, and additional lemon juice as desired.

To make the cauliflower couscous: While the chicken rests, grate the cauliflower on the coarse side of a box grater and place in a large bowl. Add the oil, lemon juice, and 1 tsp of the spice blend, and toss to combine. Fold in the pistachios and dried cherries. Season with salt and pepper.

Carve the chicken into 6 to 8 pieces. Place the cauliflower couscous on a large platter, then pile the roasted vegetables, grapes, and chicken on top, spooning some of the pan juices over it all. Serve with the chermoula and extra pan juices on the side.

STICKY ORANGE CHICKEN
with Caramelized Onions and Fennel

I have been lucky to meet many of my food idols, so I usually don't get starstruck, but I made an exception for Nigella Lawson. Out of nowhere, she reposted a picture from my book on Instagram and I nearly had a heart attack. When I had a chance to meet her a month later, I was in awe. The woman is gorgeous and gracious, and her voice is even sexier in person. I handed her the first copy of my *Anti-Inflammation Cookbook*, which was hot off the press. That night, she posted *again* on Instagram, saying she couldn't wait to "tuck in and give it a read." That's when I died and went straight to heaven. In truth, I chose to cook my way through her latest book instead. I fell in love with her version of a sheet-pan chicken—the easiest way to make an entire meal at once! Here I've put my spin on it, adding my favorite Asian ingredients. I chose fennel this time, but feel free to use bok choy, green beans, or any other veggie you'd like smothered in this sauce.

PREPARATION TIME
15 minutes
(plus 1 hour to marinate)

COOKING TIME
35–40 minutes

SERVES
4–6

½ cup [120 ml] toasted sesame oil	3 garlic cloves, minced
2 Tbsp grated orange zest plus ½ cup [120 ml] fresh orange juice	3 lb [1.3 kg] bone-in, skin-on chicken thighs
6 Tbsp [90 ml] tamari	2 large yellow onions, thinly sliced
1 Tbsp fresh lime juice	2 fennel bulbs, cored and thinly sliced, plus fennel fronds for garnish
2 Tbsp grated fresh ginger	

In a large bowl, whisk the sesame oil, orange zest and juice, tamari, lime juice, ginger, and garlic to combine. Add the chicken, onions, and fennel. Toss to coat. Marinate for at least 1 hour or up to 2 days in the refrigerator.

Preheat the oven to 400°F [200°C]. Transfer the chicken, onions, and fennel from the marinade onto a baking sheet. Arrange the chicken skin-side up on top of the onions and fennel, distributing it all evenly. Pour ½ cup [120 ml] of the marinade over the chicken (discard the remainder). Roast, turning the pan once halfway through roasting, until the skin is browned and crisp and the internal temperature of the chicken has reached 165°F [75°C], 40 to 45 minutes. Sprinkle with minced fennel fronds and serve immediately.

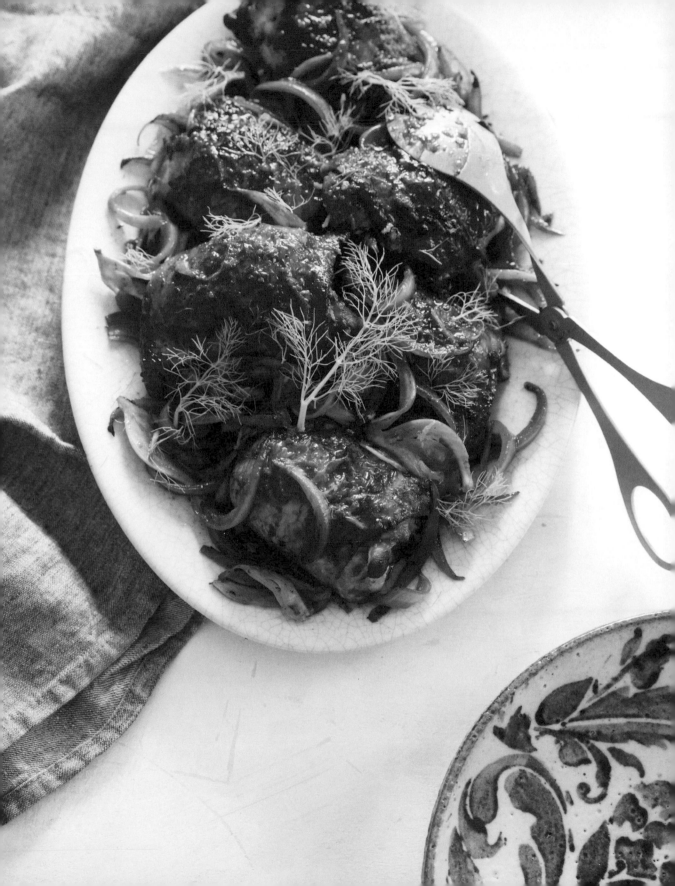

THAI CHICKEN BURGER

with Pickled Papaya Slaw

In Thai cuisine, the green papaya salad known as *som tam* has the perfect balance of the four taste sensations: sweet, sour, salty, and umami. Plus, green papaya aids digestion, soothes inflammation, and can even help fight nausea. Drawing on the flavors of som tam, I wanted to turn it into an entrée. The result? The most satiating chicken burger I've ever had, chock-full of age-defying ingredients like curry powder and coconut milk, topped with the yummy benefits of a papaya slaw. I serve mine as a lettuce wrap—no buns happening in my house—but I swear you won't even miss the bread. Ask your grocer for a green papaya if you don't see any in the store.

Make sure you buy unsweetened coconut cream for this recipe (not cream of coconut, which is a sweetened product). If canned coconut cream is unavailable, buy a can of regular coconut milk and refrigerate for several hours before opening it; you can then skim off the thick cream that has solidified at the top.

PREPARATION TIME
25 minutes

COOKING TIME
10 minutes

SERVES
4

6 oz [170 g] shredded green papaya (from 1 medium papaya)

1 red onion, thinly sliced

3 Tbsp plus 2 tsp fresh lime juice and 2 tsp grated lime zest

1 Tbsp fish sauce

6 Tbsp [90 ml] canola oil

1 stalk lemongrass, cut into ¼ in [6 mm] slices

1 lb [455 g] ground chicken thigh meat

¼ cup [60 ml] coconut cream (thick milk solids from one 14 oz [392 g] can chilled coconut milk)

½ cup [20 g] chopped fresh cilantro

2 garlic cloves, minced or grated

2 tsp grated fresh ginger

2 tsp kosher salt

1 tsp freshly ground black pepper

1 tsp ground cumin

½ cup [120 g] mayonnaise

1½ tsp curry powder

8 large leaves butter lettuce

In a medium bowl, combine the papaya, onion, 3 Tbsp of the lime juice, and the fish sauce. Cover and refrigerate until ready to use.

In a medium skillet over medium-low heat, combine the oil and lemongrass. Cook for 5 minutes, then strain the oil and reserve it, discarding the lemongrass. Set aside.

In a large bowl, stir together the ground chicken, coconut cream, cilantro, garlic, ginger, salt, pepper, cumin, lime zest, and remaining 2 tsp lime juice until thoroughly combined. Refrigerate for 20 minutes.

Meanwhile, in a small bowl, stir together the mayonnaise and curry powder. Set aside.

Form the chicken mixture into four equal patties. Heat a large skillet over medium heat. Add 3 Tbsp of the lemongrass oil, and heat until just beginning to smoke. Add the patties and cook until the internal temperature reaches 165°F [74°C], about 5 minutes per side. Add the remaining 3 Tbsp lemongrass oil when you flip the burgers.

Place each burger on a leaf of lettuce; top with curry mayonnaise and pickled papaya slaw. Top with a second lettuce leaf and serve.

PORK AND MANGO STIR-FRY

with Napa Cabbage and Toasted Almonds

I have this habit of re-creating recipes I have loved over the years, basically forgetting that I'd already written a version of it. This one's a classic. I actually have a version of it on my website and another version in my first book, and my second. (Insert my need for fish oil and other memory joggers here.) But I have to say, by starting over, I think I've made my best version yet!

I love pork as the protein, but chicken thighs or breasts work well, too. And the fact that this recipe is loaded with so many healthy ingredients in one is a total bonus. Once you prep the ingredients, it literally comes together in 7 minutes.

PREPARATION TIME
15 minutes

COOKING TIME
7 minutes

SERVES
4

1 Tbsp tamari or coconut aminos

2 tsp cornstarch

2 Tbsp fresh orange juice

2 Tbsp gluten-free flour or rice flour

1½ lb [680 g] boneless pork chops, sliced into ¼ by 2 in [6 mm by 5 cm] pieces

3 Tbsp toasted sesame oil

2 celery stalks, finely diced

4 green onions, white and light green parts only, sliced

2 garlic cloves, minced

1 tsp grated fresh ginger

1 small napa cabbage, sliced crosswise into ½ in [12 mm] pieces

2 mangoes, diced

¼ cup [40 g] coarsely chopped roasted almonds

¼ cup [8 g] chopped fresh mint

1 Tbsp black sesame seeds

In a small bowl, whisk together the tamari and cornstarch, then add the orange juice. Set aside. In another bowl, sprinkle the flour over the sliced pork and toss to coat. Set aside.

Set a large wok or nonstick skillet over medium-high heat. When the pan is hot, add 2 Tbsp of the sesame oil, then the celery. Stir-fry for 1 minute, then add the green onions and stir-fry for another minute. Add the garlic and ginger, and stir-fry until fragrant, about 1 minute. Transfer the vegetables to a plate, wipe out the pan, and add the remaining 1 Tbsp oil. When hot, add the pork and cook, stirring constantly, until the pork is just cooked through, about 2 minutes. (Depending on the size of the pan, you may need to do this in two batches.)

Return the celery mixture to the pan. Stir in the cabbage, allowing it to wilt for about 1 minute, then add the tamari and orange juice mixture and the mangoes. Remove from the heat, and stir to coat the pork and cabbage with the sauce. Fold in the almonds and mint. Sprinkle with the sesame seeds and serve immediately.

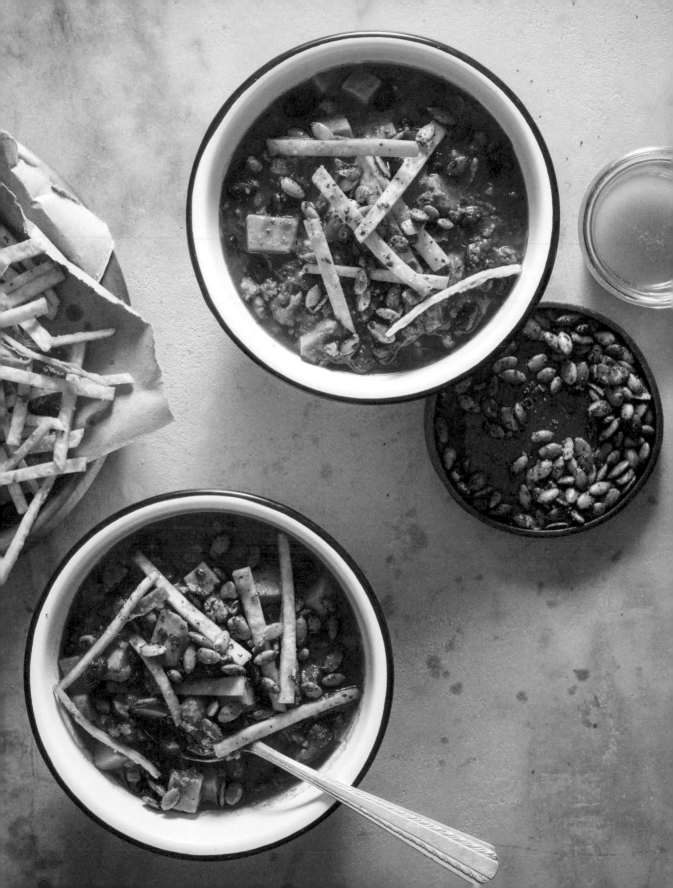

SWEET POTATO–TURKEY CHILI

with Cilantro Oil and Pepitas

There's something about chili that will never go out of style. Although I love the classic combination of ground beef, onions, red bell pepper, and beans, I'm always looking for versions with more redeeming health benefits. The sweet potatoes in this chili add loads of vitamins A, B1, B2, B6, and C, along with fiber and potassium. And I choose high-quality, organic ground turkey here, but ground beef or lamb would work just as well. With a potent fresh cilantro oil drizzled over the top, this chili recipe will leave you looking and feeling your best.

PREPARATION TIME	COOKING TIME	SERVES
20 minutes	45 minutes	6

CHILI

3 to 4 Tbsp extra-virgin olive oil	1 tsp fennel seeds
2 red onions, diced	1½ lb [680 g] ground turkey
Kosher salt	2 sweet potatoes, peeled and diced
2 Tbsp chili powder	One 28 oz [794 g] can crushed tomatoes
3 garlic cloves, minced	1½ cups [360 ml] chicken broth
1 tsp ground cumin	Two 15 oz [425 g] cans black beans or pinto beans, rinsed and drained

CILANTRO OIL

2 garlic cloves, minced	¾ cup [25 g] firmly packed cilantro leaves
2 Tbsp white wine vinegar	¼ cup [60 ml] extra-virgin olive oil
1 Tbsp sugar	Pinch of kosher salt

CONTINUED

SPICED PEPITAS

2 Tbsp olive oil	1 tsp chili powder
½ cup [60 g] pepitas	Pinch of kosher salt
1 tsp ground cumin	

FRIED TORTILLA STRIPS

2 small corn tortillas	Kosher salt
1 Tbsp olive oil	

To make the chili: In a large saucepan or Dutch oven over medium heat, warm 3 Tbsp oil. Add the onions and 2 tsp salt and cook, stirring occasionally, until soft and translucent, 5 to 8 minutes. Add the chili powder, garlic, cumin, and fennel seeds, and cook until fragrant, about 1 minute. Transfer the onions to a plate. If the pan looks dry, add 1 Tbsp oil, then add the ground turkey. Cook, breaking up the meat, until brown and just cooked through, about 5 minutes. Return the onions to the pan, and add the sweet potatoes, crushed tomatoes, and chicken broth. Bring to a boil over medium heat. Stir, reduce the heat to low, cover, and simmer until the potatoes are cooked through, 15 to 20 minutes. Stir in the beans. Season with salt.

To make the cilantro oil: While the chili is cooking, pulse the garlic in a small food processor a few times. Add the vinegar and sugar and pulse a few more times to combine. Add the cilantro and oil and process for 15 to 30 seconds, or until the mixture reaches a pourable consistency. Taste, adding salt as needed.

To make the spiced pepitas: Heat the oil in a small skillet over medium heat. Add the pepitas and toast for 2 minutes, until fragrant. Add the cumin, chili powder, and salt, and stir to coat. Cook for 1 minute, then transfer to a paper towel–lined plate.

To make the tortilla strips: Stack the corn tortillas and slice them into ¼ in [6 mm] strips. Heat a small frying pan over medium-high heat, and add the olive oil, the tortilla strips, and a generous sprinkling of salt. Cook, stirring constantly, until crisp, 1 to 2 minutes. Drain on paper towels.

Ladle the chili into bowls, drizzle with the cilantro oil, sprinkle the pepitas and tortilla strips on top, and serve.

PORK CHOPS

with Mashed Sweet Potatoes and Cranberry Sauce

If I could, I would eat the traditional Thanksgiving meal once a week. I crave those warm, fall flavors that go so well together. One of my favorite nearby restaurants—Chow in Lafayette, California—has something on the menu that always fulfills my craving: grilled chicken with mashed sweet potatoes, cranberry sauce, and Brussels sprouts loaded with bacon.

For my homemade version, I decided to use one of my favorite meats, the double-cut pork chop, and keep the sweet potatoes and cranberry sauce. Humanely and cleanly raised pork is one of the hardest meats to find, so make sure to do your research.

PREPARATION TIME
25 minutes
(plus 1½ hours to brine)

COOKING TIME
1½ hours

SERVES
4

PORK CHOPS

Kosher salt

½ cup [120 ml] maple syrup

1 tsp allspice berries

1 tsp black peppercorns

2 bay leaves

2 cups [480 ml] hot water

2 cups [280 g] ice cubes

4 double-cut, bone-in pork chops, about 3½ lb [1.6 kg]

2 Tbsp extra-virgin olive oil

Freshly ground black pepper

2 Tbsp chopped fresh rosemary, plus more for garnish

Flaked sea salt for garnish

CRANBERRY SAUCE

1 orange

12 oz [340 g] fresh cranberries

1 cinnamon stick

¼ cup [60 ml] maple syrup

½ cup [100 g] firmly packed brown sugar

Pinch of kosher salt

1 apple, finely diced

CONTINUED

MASHED SWEET POTATOES

6 medium sweet potatoes (about 2 lb [910 g], unpeeled	2 Tbsp maple syrup
	½ tsp ground ginger
2 Tbsp extra-virgin olive oil	½ tsp ground nutmeg
Kosher salt	½ tsp ground cloves
½ cup [110 g] unsalted butter (1 stick)	Freshly ground black pepper

To make the pork chops: Combine ½ cup [160 g] of kosher salt, the maple syrup, allspice berries, peppercorns, and bay leaves in a large bowl. Pour in the hot water and stir to dissolve the salt and maple syrup. Add the ice cubes, and stir until melted, with the liquid no longer warm to the touch. Place the pork chops in the brine and cover. Refrigerate for at least 1½ hours or up to overnight.

To make the cranberry sauce: Peel the zest from the orange in wide strips, then juice the orange. In a small saucepan over medium heat, combine the orange zest and juice, cranberries, cinnamon stick, maple syrup, sugar, and salt. Cook, stirring occasionally, until the cranberries burst and the sauce thickens, about 30 minutes. Remove from the heat; discard the orange zest and cinnamon stick. Stir in the apple and set aside.

To make the mashed sweet potatoes: Preheat the oven to 400°F [200°C]. Place the sweet potatoes on a parchment-lined baking sheet. Drizzle with the oil and sprinkle with salt. Roast until very tender, about 45 minutes. Let stand at room temperature until cool enough to handle. Remove the peels, and use a ricer or handheld masher to mash the sweet potatoes into a saucepan or small Dutch oven. In a small saucepan over medium heat, melt the butter. Cook, swirling frequently, until the butter browns and smells nutty, 6 to 8 minutes. Pour the brown butter into the mashed sweet potatoes, along with the maple syrup, ginger, nutmeg, and cloves, and stir to combine. Season with kosher salt and pepper. Cover and keep warm.

While the sweet potatoes are roasting, remove the pork chops from the brine and pat dry. Heat a grill pan over high heat. Drizzle the pork chops with the oil, and season generously on both sides with kosher salt, pepper, and the chopped rosemary. Arrange the pork chops on the grill pan, and cook until charred and golden brown on both sides, about 5 minutes per side. Transfer the pork chops to a baking sheet, and place in the oven with the sweet potatoes; cook to your preferred doneness, about 145°F [63°C] for medium-rare, 10 to 15 minutes. Remove from the oven and let rest for 5 minutes.

Warm the cranberry sauce gently over low heat. Divide the mashed sweet potatoes among individual plates. Slice the pork chops and arrange over the mashed sweet potatoes; sprinkle with extra chopped rosemary and flaked sea salt. Spoon some of the cranberry sauce on the side and serve.

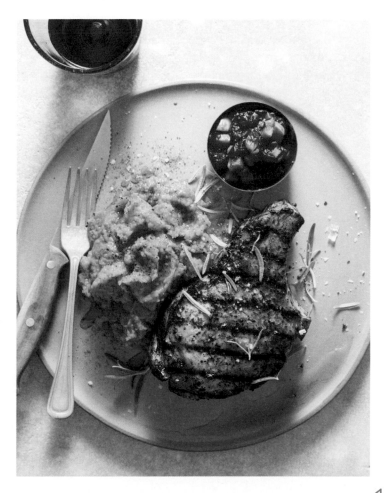

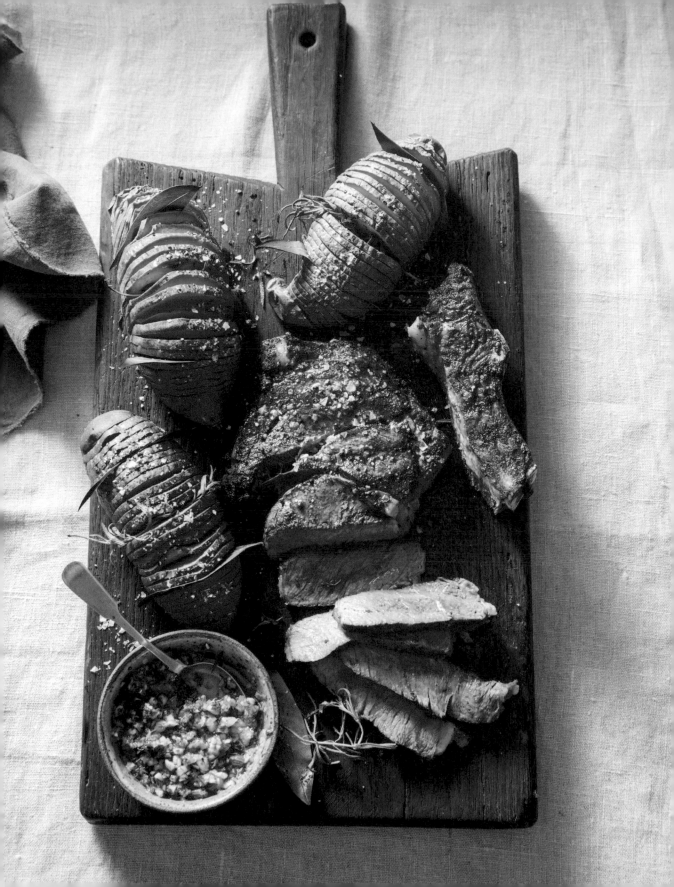

GRILLED RIB EYES

with Hasselback Sweet Potatoes and Preserved Lemon Gremolata

The benefits of consuming organic grass-fed meat rather than conventional grain-fed meat are remarkable. When cattle are given a diet of grass instead of corn and grain, their meat actually has higher levels of omega-3 (the anti-inflammatory fat) and lower levels of omega-6 (the pro-inflammatory fat), making it a much healthier choice for us. In addition, certified organic meats are free of hormones and antibiotic compounds that can cause problems with our endocrine systems and potentially cause hormone-dependent cancers. Many grocers are now labeling their meat and showing you what the cattle are fed. My optimal resource is Belcampo Meats out of the Bay Area, but Whole Foods Market and many others are doing a wonderful job offering grass-fed versions of our favorite cuts, too.

The word *Hasselback* refers to the Swedish recipe *Hasselbackspotatis*, where potatoes are cut about halfway through into thin slices, and then butter, bread crumbs, and almonds are added on top. I keep the method of slicing them thinly, but change up the ingredients for a healthier spin. They're delicious with this herby, punchy gremolata, but for the holidays they would be equally as delicious drizzled with a little melted butter, brown sugar, cinnamon, ginger, and nutmeg. For a dramatic effect, you can also nestle fresh herbs into the sweet potatoes before roasting them. No matter which ingredients you choose to add, they will look amazing and cook evenly.

PREPARATION TIME
10 minutes

COOKING TIME
50–60 minutes

SERVES
4

---

2 bone-in rib-eye steaks, about 1½ lb [680 g] each

4 sweet potatoes, about 8 oz [225 g] each

Extra-virgin olive oil

Kosher salt

Freshly ground black pepper

Preserved Lemon Gremolata (page 221)

One hour before serving, remove the steaks from the refrigerator to allow them to come to room temperature.

Using a sharp knife, cut each sweet potato crosswise into ⅛ in [3 mm] slices, cutting only three-fourths of the way through the potatoes so they stay intact.

CONTINUED

To prepare the potatoes in the oven: Preheat the oven to 425°F [220°C]. Place the cut potatoes, sliced-side up, on a foil-lined baking sheet. Drizzle with oil, and season generously with salt and pepper. Roast until the potatoes are browned on the outside and tender in the center, 50 to 60 minutes.

To prepare the potatoes on the grill: Prepare a grill for direct cooking over medium-high heat, 400°F [200°C]. Grease the grill grate lightly. Place the cut potatoes on a grill-safe roasting pan. Drizzle with oil, and season generously with salt and pepper. Place the pan on the grill, then cover the grill. Roast until the potatoes are browned on the outside and tender in the center, 50 to 60 minutes. Remove the potatoes from the grill or transfer to the warming section of the grill.

Rub each steak with oil, and sprinkle salt and pepper generously over each side. Place the steaks on the grill and cook, allowing each side to sear, until the internal temperature of the steak reaches 130°F [55°C] for medium-rare, 4 to 5 minutes per side. Remove the steaks from the grill, and let rest for 10 minutes.

Slice the steaks against the grain. Place the potatoes and sliced steak on a platter. Drizzle a spoonful of the gremolata over each sweet potato and serve, passing the remaining gremolata at the table.

STEAK TACOS

with Cabbage Slaw, Mango Salsa, and Chipotle Mayonnaise

I'll put pretty much anything in a corn tortilla and call it a taco. I'm happiest when somebody brings a basket of tortillas to my table so I can pile my eggs, grilled meat, pickled veggies, or beans in one for breakfast, lunch, or dinner. Over the years, I've developed a dozen different taco recipes, but this one takes top honors. You can do as much or as little as you'd like for this recipe. No time to make the mango salsa? You can buy some already made. Also, the meat can marinate overnight, and the cabbage slaw can be made a day in advance, too.

If you're looking for an alternative to steak, the marinade is delicious on chicken, too. For a vegetarian version, grilled mushrooms, peppers, or squash would all be delicious alternatives.

PREPARATION TIME
45 minutes
(plus 1 hour to marinate)

COOKING TIME
10 minutes

SERVES
4

STEAK TACOS

¼ cup [60 ml] fresh orange juice	Kosher salt
3 Tbsp fresh lime juice	Freshly ground black pepper
1 chipotle chile in adobo plus 1 Tbsp adobo sauce	1 lb [455 g] skirt steak
	Olive oil
2 Tbsp honey	Eight to twelve 6 in [15 cm] corn tortillas
2 garlic cloves, grated	
2 tsp ground cumin	

CABBAGE SLAW

½ head purple cabbage, thinly sliced	2 tsp honey
2 Tbsp extra-virgin olive oil	Kosher salt
2 tsp fresh lime juice	Freshly ground black pepper

CONTINUED

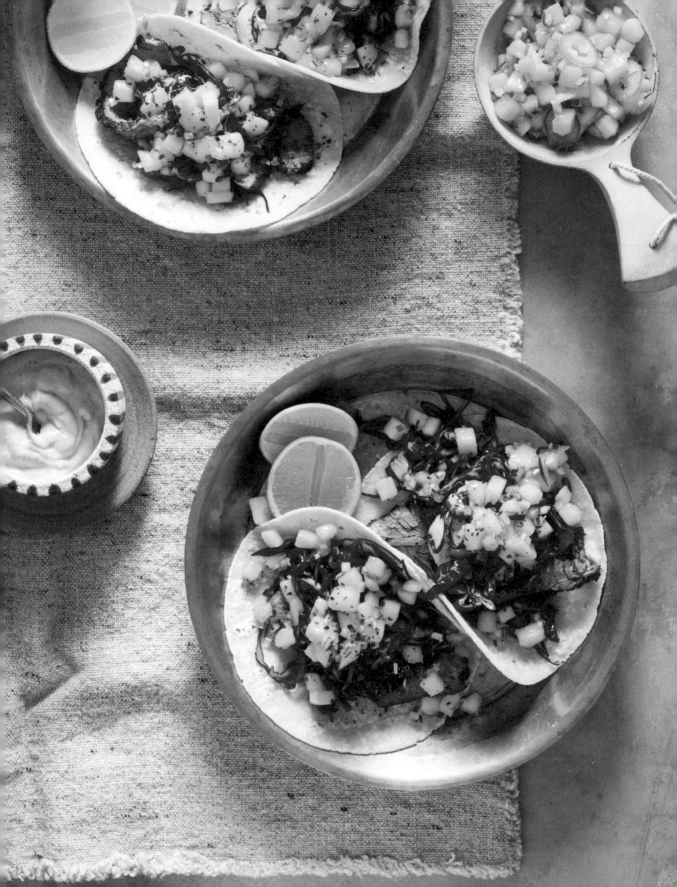

MANGO SALSA

2 mangoes, diced	1 jalapeño, diced
1 red onion, diced	1 Tbsp fresh lime juice

CHIPOTLE MAYONNAISE

½ cup [120 g] mayonnaise	2 tsp adobo sauce

To make the steak tacos: In a large bowl, combine the orange juice, lime juice, chipotle chile and adobo sauce, honey, garlic, and cumin. Season with salt and pepper. Add the steak and turn to coat with the marinade. Refrigerate for 1 hour.

To make the cabbage slaw: Combine the cabbage, oil, lime juice, and honey in a medium bowl, and season with salt and pepper; toss to coat. Refrigerate until ready to use, at least 20 minutes.

To make the mango salsa: Combine the mangoes, onion, jalapeño, and lime juice in a medium bowl, and toss to coat. Refrigerate until ready to use, at least 20 minutes.

To make the chipotle mayonnaise: Mix the mayonnaise and adobo sauce together in a small bowl.

Heat a large skillet or grill pan over medium-high heat, and brush with oil. Sear the steak until the internal temperature reaches 130°F [55°C] for medium-rare, about 3 minutes per side. Transfer the steak to a cutting board, and let rest for 10 minutes. Meanwhile, heat the tortillas on the skillet or grill pan over medium heat until warmed. Cut the steak into ½ in [12 mm] slices. Fill each tortilla with about 2 oz [55 g] of steak, a dollop of chipotle mayo, and a spoonful each of cabbage slaw and mango salsa. Serve immediately.

COCONUT GINGER SEA BASS
in PARCHMENT
with King Trumpet Mushrooms and Bok Choy

When I write cookbooks, I tend to isolate myself, relying on my own instincts to develop the recipes before sharing them with friends and family for feedback. During this book's creation, I opened myself up for feedback a little sooner, and what happened? Magic! Belle English, an amazing recipe developer and test cook, suggested the addition of coconut milk, and it sang! With the health benefits of ginger, garlic, mushrooms, bok choy, and coconut milk all in one place, this recipe will make you feel as great as it tastes. Also, serving the fish in its parchment is always a total showstopper. No one has to know it's a piece of cake.

If you like starch with your meal, serve each packet with a side of brown rice. You can let all of the amazing flavors from the coconut milk and sea bass absorb into the rice. Perfection.

PREPARATION TIME
30 minutes

COOKING TIME
20 minutes

SERVES
4

Four 4 oz [115 g] sea bass fillets

Kosher salt

Freshly ground black pepper

¼ cup [60 ml] toasted sesame oil

¼ cup [60 ml] tamari

¼ cup [60 ml] coconut milk

1 tsp grated lime zest plus 2 Tbsp fresh lime juice, plus lime wedges for serving

1 Tbsp grated fresh ginger

---

2 tsp honey

2 garlic cloves, minced or grated

8 oz [225 g] King Trumpet mushrooms, thinly sliced lengthwise

2 heads baby bok choy, cut into ¼ in [6 mm] slices on the bias

3 green onions, thinly sliced, dark green parts reserved for garnish

Toasted sesame seeds for garnish (optional)

Preheat the oven to 400°F [200°C]. Cut four pieces of parchment, each 18 in [46 cm] long.

Season the fish with a small pinch each of salt and pepper. In a medium mixing bowl, whisk together the sesame oil, tamari, coconut milk, lime zest and juice, ginger, honey, and garlic. Reserve 6 Tbsp [90 ml] of the marinade. Add the fish to the remaining marinade and toss to coat. Cover and marinate at room temperature for 20 minutes.

CONTINUED

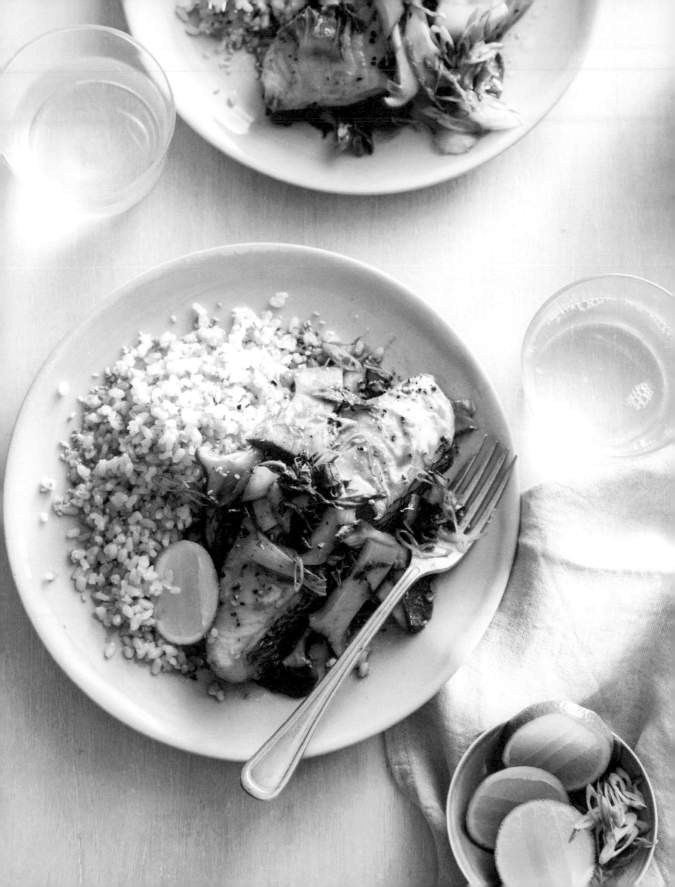

Combine the mushrooms, bok choy, and green onion whites in a bowl. Season lightly with salt and pepper. Drizzle with the reserved marinade and toss to coat.

Place a handful of the mushroom mixture in the center of a piece of parchment. Place a fish fillet on top, and add another handful of mushrooms. Bring the long sides of the paper together, and fold the top edges down together to create a 1 in [2.5 cm] seam, then continue to fold down tightly over the fish and vegetables. Twist the open ends of the parchment in opposite directions to prevent steam from escaping. Place the packet on a baking sheet. Repeat the process with the remaining ingredients and parchment. Bake until the packets are browned and have puffed up, about 15 minutes.

Transfer each packet to a plate and let stand for 5 minutes. Using sharp scissors, cut an X into the center of each packet, and carefully pull back the parchment. Sprinkle with green onion greens and sesame seeds, if using. Serve immediately with lime wedges.

TUNA POKE

with Miso Mayonnaise and Pickled Cucumber

Tuna tartare was all the rage when I moved to San Francisco in 1994, and it's been on menus ever since! And with good reason: the silky texture of high-quality tuna contrasted with the crunch of nuts or cucumbers is highly addictive. The best part about tuna tartare is that it's incredibly versatile. You can take it from Latin to Asian-inspired simply by changing the oil or acid you choose. This version is influenced by the Hawaiian tuna poke bowl. Sesame oil and tamari lend depth, and the cucumber, green onions, and macadamia nuts give it crunch and contrast. If you want, you can skip the rice paper and mayo, but with it, it is the most decadent, perfect poke you'll ever taste.

PREPARATION TIME
20 minutes

COOKING TIME
5 minutes

SERVES
4–6 as a meal (or 12 as an appetizer)

PICKLED CUCUMBER

½ English cucumber, thinly sliced	3 Tbsp packed brown sugar
½ cup [120 ml] water	1 Tbsp kosher salt
½ cup [120 ml] rice vinegar	

MISO MAYONNAISE

1 Tbsp miso paste	¾ cup [180 g] mayonnaise
1 Tbsp hot water	

CONTINUED

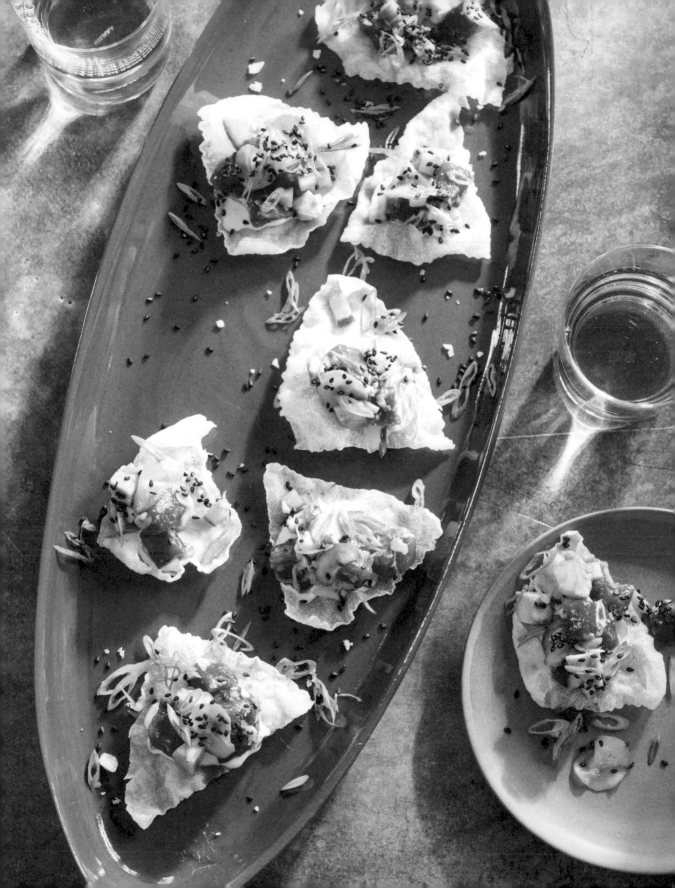

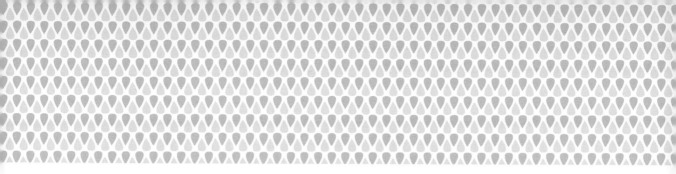

RICE CRISPS

Canola oil, for frying	Kosher salt
10 spring roll rice wrappers, cut into sixths	

TUNA TARTARE

1 lb [455 g] fresh ahi-grade tuna, cut into ½ in [12 mm] dice	2 Tbsp tamari
1 avocado, cut into ½ inch [12 mm] dice	2 Tbsp mirin
½ cup [80 g] macadamia nuts, chopped	1 Tbsp toasted sesame oil
3 green onions, white and light green parts only, thinly sliced	Black sesame seeds for garnish

To make the pickled cucumber: Place the sliced cucumber in a ceramic or glass bowl. In a small saucepan over high heat, combine the water, vinegar, sugar, and salt and bring to a boil. Stir to dissolve the salt and sugar, then pour the liquid over the cucumber. Let stand until cooled to room temperature, then cover and refrigerate until ready to use.

To make the miso mayonnaise: In a small bowl, whisk together the miso paste and hot water until smooth. Stir in the mayonnaise. Set aside.

To make the rice crisps: Fill a medium saucepan two-thirds full with canola oil and heat to 350°F [180°C]. Carefully place a few rice wrapper triangles in the oil until they turn white and puff, about 30 seconds. Transfer to a paper towel–lined plate, and sprinkle with salt. Repeat with the remaining wrappers.

To make the tuna tartare: In a large mixing bowl, gently fold together the tuna, avocado, macadamia nuts, and 2 Tbsp of the green onions. Drain the pickled cucumber slices from their liquid, and add the slices to the bowl. Add the tamari, mirin, and sesame oil, and gently fold to coat the tuna mixture.

Place 1 tsp of the miso mayonnaise on a rice crisp, then top with tuna tartare. Repeat with the remaining crisps, mayonnaise, and tuna. Arrange them on a platter, then garnish with black sesame seeds and the remaining green onions. Serve.

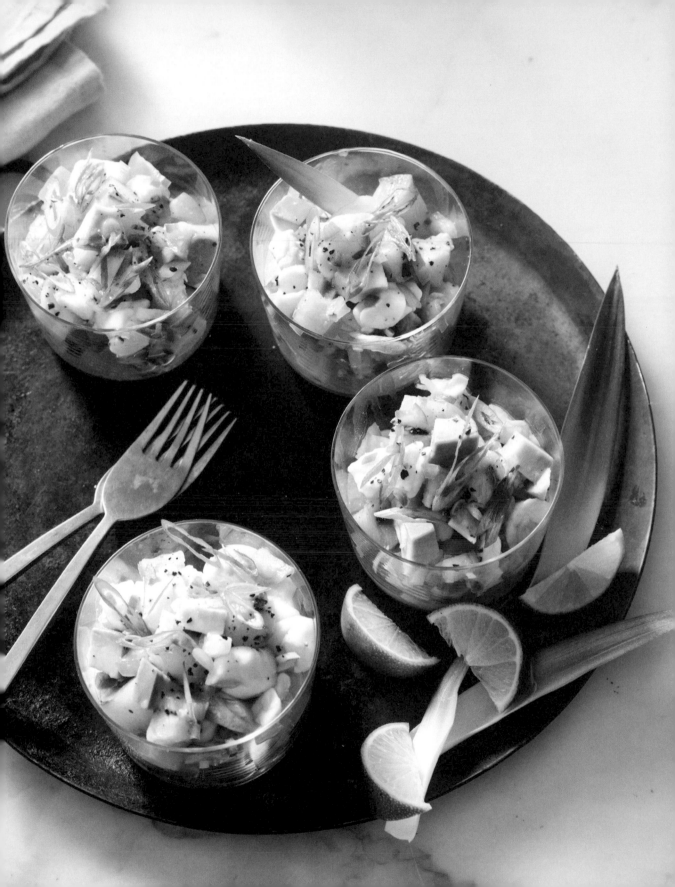

CEVICHE

with Grilled Pineapple, Tomatillos, and Jalapeño

Ceviche is my magical recipe for entertaining. It seems kinda sexy, being raw fish that gets "cooked" with citrus. Plus, the core ingredients in ceviche, like citrus, fruit, fish, herbs, and chiles, are all nutritional powerhouses.

In this rendition, I chose grilled pineapple to add a little smokiness, but you can certainly use raw diced pineapple or mango if you're short on time. One important tip: Do not let the ceviche sit overnight. The longer it sits in the citrus, the more the fish "cooks," which changes the texture of the dish. So, prep the ingredients anytime on the day you're serving it, then put them together thirty to sixty minutes beforehand, and you'll be thrilled with the results.

If you're serving this as an appetizer, sliced jicama, taro chips, or fresh corn chips are great vehicles for scooping up the ceviche!

PREPARATION TIME
40 minutes
(plus 30 minutes to chill)

SERVES
6–10

Olive oil

1 pineapple, peeled, cored, and cut into ½ in [12 mm] slices

1 lb [455 g] halibut or other firm-fleshed white fish, cut into ½ in [12 mm] pieces

½ cup [120 ml] fresh lime juice

2 green onions, white and light green parts only, thinly sliced

1 tsp kosher salt

1 jalapeño, seeded and minced

2 tomatillos, outer skin removed, cut into ¼ in [6 mm] pieces

1 avocado, diced

Freshly ground pepper

Heat a grill pan over medium-high heat and brush with oil. Grill the pineapple until soft and slightly translucent, about 10 minutes. Transfer to a plate to cool completely, then cut into ½ in [12 mm] pieces.

Put the halibut, lime juice, green onions, and salt in a shallow ceramic or glass dish. Stir to coat the fish with the lime juice, then add the jalapeño. Cover and refrigerate for 30 to 60 minutes, allowing the citrus to "cook" the fish. The fish will be opaque when ready.

Gently fold in the tomatillos, avocado, and pineapple. Season with salt and pepper, and serve immediately.

PAN-SEARED SCALLOPS

with Citrusy Corn Succotash

To me, scallops feel like a total luxury food, but believe it or not, they have huge health benefits. Three ounces [85 g] of scallops have 20 grams of protein and less than 100 calories, and they're loaded with magnesium, potassium, and vitamin B12—all key components to aging well. You won't see me using corn a lot, as it's almost impossible to find organic corn that hasn't been sprayed with all kinds of nonsense. When I find it, I prepare it simply so you get nothing but the fresh taste of sweet, crunchy, summery corn.

PREPARATION TIME
25 minutes

COOKING TIME
15 minutes

SERVES
4

---

16 large scallops, about 1½ lb [680 g]

Kosher salt

2 Tbsp olive oil

2 garlic cloves, smashed and peeled

2 tsp grated lime zest plus 2 Tbsp fresh lime juice

2 Tbsp water

3 Tbsp unsalted butter

Kernels from 2 ears corn

1 cup [170 g] cherry tomatoes, sliced

3 Tbsp chopped chives

Rinse the scallops under cold water. Pat dry with a paper towel until they are completely dry. Sprinkle both sides of the scallops with salt.

In a large skillet over low heat, heat the oil and garlic. Cook until the garlic is browned and fragrant, about 2 minutes, then use a slotted spoon to remove it. Increase the heat to medium-high. When the pan is very hot and the oil is shimmering, add the scallops, making sure not to overcrowd the pan. Sear the scallops until they develop a golden crust, about 2 minutes, then flip and sear until they are barely opaque, about 2 minutes more. Transfer to a paper towel–lined plate.

Wipe any burned areas on the pan, then return to medium-high heat. Add 1 Tbsp of the lime juice and the water to the pan and cook, scraping up any browned bits. Add the butter, corn, tomatoes, lime zest, and a generous pinch of salt. Cook until the tomatoes give off their juices and the sauce thickens, about 4 minutes. Stir in the chives. Taste, adding more salt and lime juice if necessary. Spoon a generous helping of the corn succotash onto individual plates, top with the scallops, and serve.

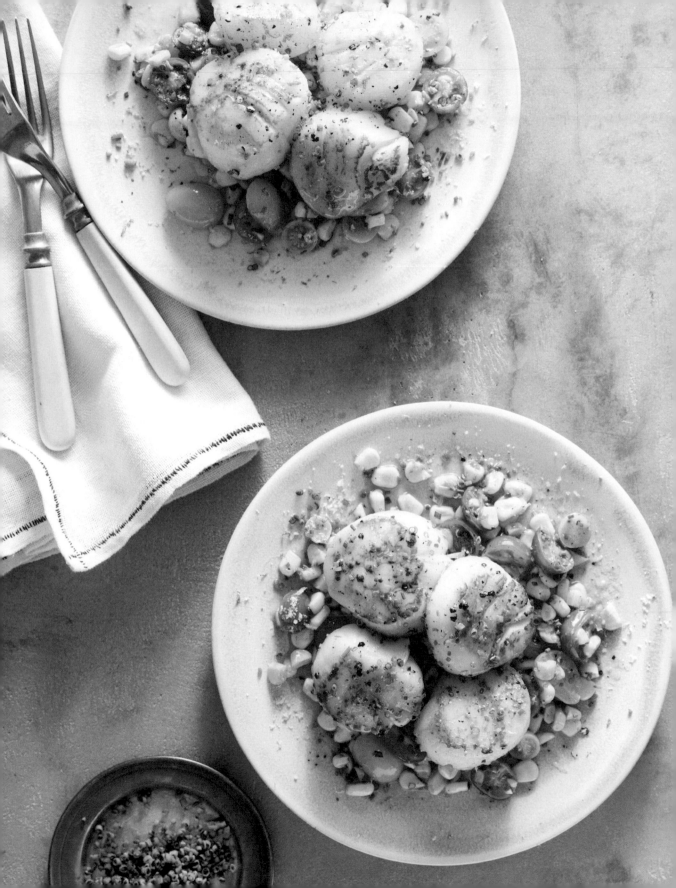

WHOLE-ROASTED FISH

with Currant Brown Butter Sauce

Roasting a whole fish looks intimidating, but I'm telling you it's one of the most forgiving cooking methods ever. When you roast anything on the bone, the flesh is more flavorful and more tender. When you buy a whole fish, the eyes should be clear, and the fish should smell like the ocean. If it smells "fishy," that means it's old. You can ask your fishmonger to gut and scale your fish so it's ready to go.

When purchasing whole fish, plan on 1 lb [455 g] per person. I developed this recipe with a 4 lb [1.8 kg] arctic char, but it works really well with four 1 lb [455 g] branzino, too.

PREPARATION TIME
15 minutes

COOKING TIME
10–40 minutes

SERVES
4

CURRANT BROWN BUTTER SAUCE

¼ cup [55 g] unsalted butter	3 Tbsp currants or raisins
¼ cup [60 ml] extra-virgin olive oil	1 Tbsp capers
½ fennel bulb, cored and diced	⅓ cup [55 g] toasted pine nuts
Kosher salt	2 Tbsp chopped fresh mint
2 garlic cloves, peeled and thinly sliced	Freshly ground pepper
1 tsp grated lemon zest plus 1 Tbsp fresh lemon juice	

FISH

4 lb [1.8 kg] whole bone-in fish, gutted and scaled	½ fennel bulb, cored and thinly sliced
Extra-virgin olive oil	2 garlic cloves, thinly sliced
Kosher salt	4 sprigs fresh parsley, plus chopped parsley for garnish
1 lemon, sliced into ¼ in [6 mm] rounds	4 sprigs fresh mint, plus chopped mint for garnish

To make the brown butter sauce: In a large skillet over medium-low heat, heat the butter until it begins to turn brown and emit a nutty fragrance, about 3 minutes. Immediately add the oil, then add the fennel and a generous pinch of salt. Cook until the fennel is soft, stirring frequently, 5 to 8 minutes. Add the garlic and cook until fragrant, about 1 minute. Stir in the lemon zest and juice, currants, and capers, and cook until the sauce has reduced slightly and the lemon juice mellows, about 2 minutes. Set aside.

To make the fish: Preheat the oven to 400°F [200°C], or prepare a grill for direct cooking over medium-high heat, 400°F [200°C].

Rinse the fish and pat it thoroughly to dry inside and out. Lightly brush the outside and inside of the fish with oil, then sprinkle salt evenly over the inside flesh. Layer the lemon slices, fennel, garlic, and herbs evenly inside the fish. Place the oiled fish on a baking sheet, making sure it is grill-proof if grilling.

Place the sheet in the oven or on the grill. Cook (covered if using a grill) until the flesh looks opaque and flakes easily when poked with a fork, 20 to 30 minutes in the oven or 25 to 35 minutes on the grill.

Transfer the fish to a platter, and let rest for 10 minutes. While the fish is resting, rewarm the sauce, then stir in the pine nuts and mint, and season with salt and pepper. Pour a small amount of the sauce over the whole fish, and sprinkle with the chopped herbs. Serve, passing the remaining sauce at the table.

COCONUT THAI PRAWNS

with Turmeric and Ginger

I'm lucky to have some incredible chefs and cooks on speed dial. For Thai food, I call on my friend Max Borthwick. Max and his mom Toi created a line of Thai sauces using the best ingredients around, called Thaifusions. Their sauces aren't strictly Thai, but you always know that's where they started. For this recipe, Max encouraged me to seek out fingerroot instead of traditional ginger. As I researched it, I learned that fingerroot contains antioxidant, anti-inflammatory, and anticancer properties that combat gastrointestinal issues, help balance yeast in our bodies, and keep us feeling energized. Here I combine it with another anti-inflammatory ingredient—turmeric—to create a delicious, one-of-a-kind marinade. Substitute chicken thighs or a thick, white-fleshed fish like halibut, cut into 1 in [2.5 cm] cubes, or shrimp, for the prawns if you prefer.

PREPARATION TIME
15 minutes
(plus 4 hours to marinate)

COOKING TIME
10 minutes

SERVES
6

One 13.5 oz [398 ml] can coconut milk

2 Tbsp fish sauce

2 Tbsp green curry paste

2 Tbsp packed brown sugar

2 Tbsp grated fresh fingerroot or ginger

2 Tbsp fresh lime juice

2 tsp ground turmeric

1 tsp kosher salt

½ tsp freshly ground black pepper

2 lb [910 g] large prawns or colossal shrimp (about 24 prawns or shrimp), shelled

8 long wooden skewers

One 14 oz [396 g] box stir-fry rice noodles

2 Tbsp toasted sesame oil

3 garlic cloves, minced

Fresh cilantro leaves for garnish

Combine the coconut milk, fish sauce, curry paste, brown sugar, fingerroot, lime juice, turmeric, salt, and pepper in a large saucepan. Cook over medium heat, whisking frequently, for about 3 minutes. Set aside 1 cup [240 ml] of the marinade. Transfer the remaining warm marinade to a heatproof bowl, and refrigerate until cool. Add the prawns to the chilled marinade, and toss to coat. Refrigerate for at least 4 hours or up to 8 hours.

One hour before serving, soak the wooden skewers in water. Thirty minutes before serving, remove the prawns from the refrigerator. Thread the prawns onto the skewers, dividing them evenly.

Prepare a grill for cooking over medium-high heat, 400°F [200°C]. Grease the grill grate lightly, then place the skewers on the grill. Cook, turning once, until the prawns are pink and slightly browned, 4 to 6 minutes total.

As the prawns come off the grill, prepare the rice noodles according to the package instructions. Drain and rinse under cool water. In a large skillet over medium heat, warm the sesame oil. Add the garlic and sauté until fragrant, about 1 minute. Add the rice noodles and toss to coat.

Warm the reserved marinade in a small saucepan over medium-low heat. Arrange the prawns over the rice noodles, drizzle with the warm marinade, and garnish with cilantro leaves. Serve immediately.

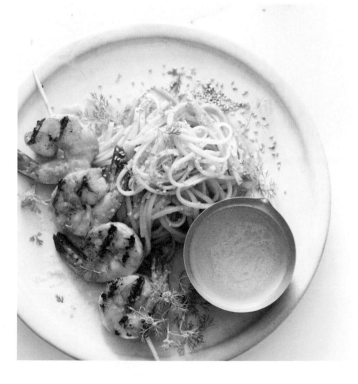

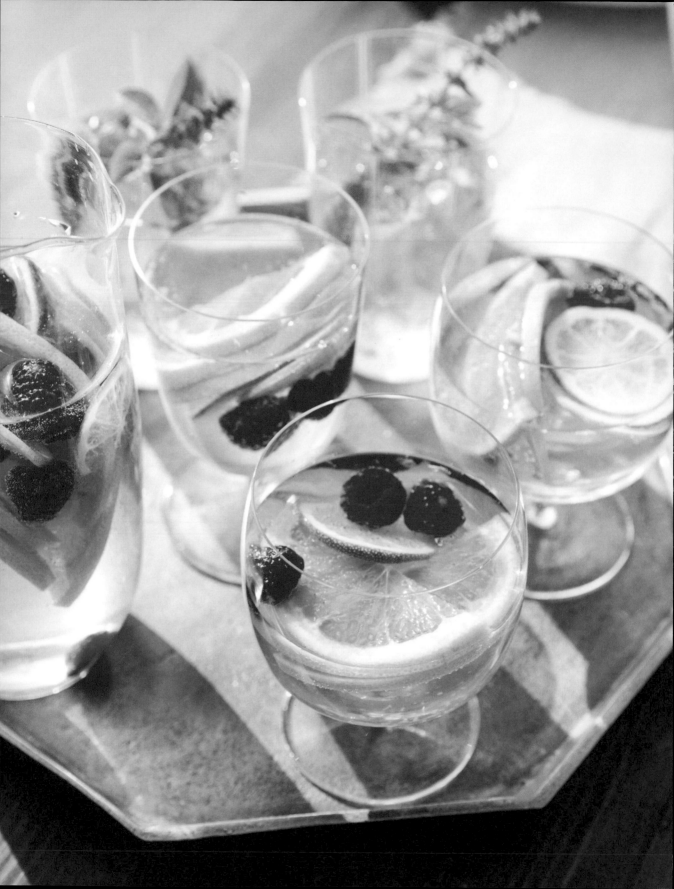

chapter

4

SWEETS, TREATS, AND COCKTAILS

Life is too short not to eat dessert. But sugar has certainly taken over our lives in a way we never could have expected, hiding in ketchup, salad dressing, dairy products, and pretty much anything else that is boxed or canned. We are consuming excessive amounts of sugar without even getting to dessert.

My goal is to cook meals that are made with real ingredients and then treat myself to desserts that are so satisfying I don't crave excessive amounts of them.

In this chapter, you'll see me use a little dairy—nothing makes a chocolate ganache tart taste better than some real cream—as well as modest amounts of sugar (I strongly recommend natural cane sugar) and other sweeteners. I still steer completely away from gluten, as I can't tolerate it at all, but you can certainly use regular flour where I call for gluten-free.

These are the absolute best versions of these recipes that I have ever developed, and I'm proud that each one has a few redeeming health qualities, so enjoy! After all, a life well lived involves pleasure—and moments of indulgence.

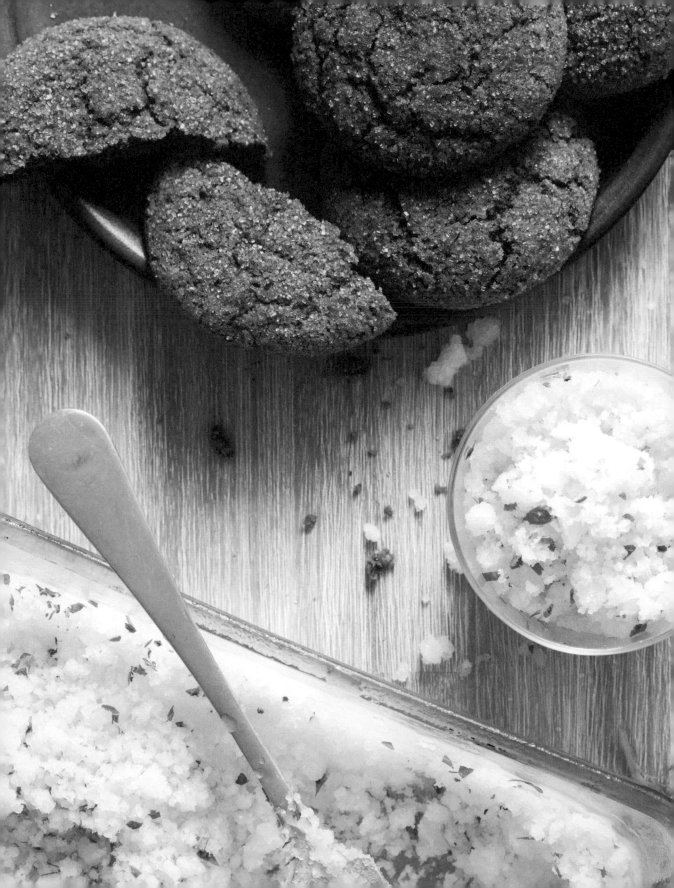

GLUTEN-FREE GINGER MOLASSES COOKIES

Since giving up gluten, there are only a few things I really miss: deep-dish and thin-crust pizzas, freshly baked bread, and cookies—I mean really good cookies. One day in the test kitchen, I was lamenting the fact I hadn't had a good ginger molasses cookie in years. Our test cook, Belle English, jumped at the challenge. Her results were pure heaven. These cookies might not be considered health food, but I promise, they're a pretty awesome version of what can be a really processed cookie. The almond flour and coconut oil only add to the flavor of this chewy, fluffy masterpiece.

PREPARATION TIME
15 minutes
(plus 20 minutes for chilling the dough)

COOKING TIME
11 minutes

MAKES
12 cookies

¼ cup [40 g] unrefined coconut oil, melted and cooled

¾ cup [150 g] sugar

3 Tbsp molasses

1 egg plus 1 yolk

2 tsp vanilla extract

½ cup [55 g] almond flour

1 cup [160 g] gluten-free flour, such as Cup4Cup or Bob's Red Mill

1 tsp kosher salt

1 tsp ground ginger

½ tsp ground cinnamon

½ tsp ground allspice

½ tsp baking soda

Preheat the oven to 350°F [180°C]. Line two baking sheets with parchment paper.

In a large bowl, whisk the coconut oil, ½ cup [100 g] of the sugar, the molasses, egg and yolk, and vanilla until the mixture is cohesive. Add both flours, the salt, ginger, cinnamon, allspice, and baking soda, and fold to combine until no streaks of flour remain. Refrigerate the dough for 20 minutes.

Place the remaining ¼ cup [50 g] sugar in a small bowl. Scoop 2 rounded Tbsp of dough and roll into a ball. Roll in the sugar, pressing gently to adhere, and place on a prepared baking sheet. Repeat with the remaining dough, spacing the balls at least 2 in [5 cm] apart. Bake until the cookies are lightly browned, 9 to 11 minutes. Let cool on the baking sheets for 10 minutes before transferring to a wire rack to cool completely.

STONE FRUIT AND BERRY CRISP

This is the perfect example of a dessert that is a delicious way to end a meal, yet is full of redeeming qualities, like oats, antioxidant-rich fruit, and almond meal. I *love* fruit crisps, and one of the things I like the most is that they're totally versatile. In summer, I load them up with stone fruits like peaches and plums. In the fall, apples and pears win out. I love to throw in some berries to balance things out. Basically, make it your own.

PREPARATION TIME
20 minutes

COOKING TIME
45 minutes

SERVES
8

---

2 cups [200 g] gluten-free rolled oats, such as Bob's Red Mill

½ cup [100 g] firmly packed brown sugar

2 tsp ground cinnamon

½ tsp ground ginger

½ tsp kosher salt

½ cup [110 g] unsalted butter, cold, cut into 16 pieces

---

3 lb [1.4 kg] stone fruit, such as peaches, plums, nectarines, or apricots, sliced

12 oz [340 g] berries, such as raspberries

1½ Tbsp fresh lemon juice

1 Tbsp cornstarch

1 Tbsp granulated sugar

1 tsp vanilla extract

Preheat the oven to 400°F [200°C].

Combine the oats, brown sugar, cinnamon, ginger, and salt in a large bowl. Add the cold butter and, using a pastry blender or fork, cut the butter into the mixture until pea-size clumps form. Set aside in the freezer.

Put the fruit in a large bowl. Sprinkle in the lemon juice, cornstarch, granulated sugar, and vanilla. Toss gently just until the cornstarch is dissolved and the fruit is evenly coated.

Pour the fruit into a 9 by 13 in [23 by 33 cm] baking dish and spread the oat mixture evenly over the top. Cover with aluminum foil and bake for 20 minutes. Remove the foil and bake until the fruit is bubbling and the top is browned, 20 to 25 minutes more. Let cool for 15 minutes before serving.

GREEK FROZEN YOGURT

with Luxardo Cherries and Dark Chocolate Chunks

I love the Greek frozen yogurt I get at Souvla, a Greek fast-casual restaurant that is taking the Bay Area by storm. The owner, a French Laundry alum, serves up the most incredible roasted lamb, chicken, and sweet potato sandwiches and salads, and his frozen yogurt is to die for. While I wait for them to open a location in my neck of the woods, I decided to blend up my own version. The best part? Greek yogurt only needs to churn for ten to thirty minutes to get the perfect creamy consistency. Studded with Luxardo cherries (I like to think that the Italian gods made these just for me) and swirled with a bunch of dark chocolate chunks, this frozen yogurt is the ultimate finish to a delicious Mediterranean meal, or the perfect snack when you feel like treating yourself.

PREPARATION TIME
10 minutes

COOKING TIME
10–45 minutes

SERVES
6

---

32 oz [910 g] whole-milk Greek yogurt

1/3 cup [65 g] sugar

1 Tbsp fresh lemon juice

1/4 cup [60 g] Luxardo maraschino cherries in their syrup, plus more for topping

1/2 cup [90 g] dark chocolate chunks or chips, such as Guittard

---

Place the yogurt in a fine-mesh strainer over a large bowl, and let drain for 2 hours. Discard any liquid that collects. (If short on time, simply spoon any excess liquid off the top of the yogurt before continuing. The more you drain the yogurt, the creamier it will be.)

Place the drained yogurt in a large bowl, and whisk in the sugar and lemon juice. Transfer the yogurt to an ice-cream machine, and freeze according to the manufacturer's instructions. After churning for 5 minutes, add the cherries, syrup, and chocolate chunks. Check the machine often, and churn until the yogurt is just frozen, 10 to 45 minutes, depending on the machine. Serve immediately, or place in an airtight container in the freezer for a few hours. To serve, scoop into bowls and spoon some Luxardo cherries and syrup over the top.

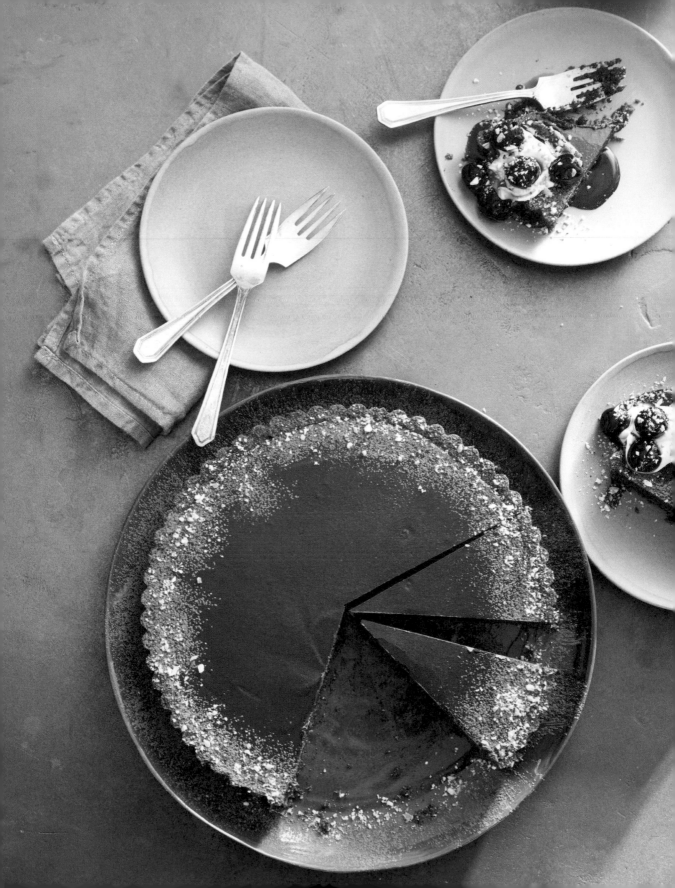

CHOCOLATE GANACHE TART

with Grand Marnier

In my effort to constantly strike a balance between health and deliciousness, I've created a tart that is better for you than most store-bought versions, but incredibly decadent. Guittard chocolate is my absolute favorite in this recipe.

PREPARATION TIME
15 minutes
(plus 4 hours to cool and set)

COOKING TIME
20 minutes

SERVES
12

2 cups [220 g] blanched almond flour

⅓ cup [40 g] cocoa powder, such as Guittard or Droste, plus more for garnish

6 Tbsp [85 g] unsalted butter, melted and slightly cooled

⅓ cup [80 ml] maple syrup

Kosher salt

1 lb [455 g] high-quality dark chocolate chips or chunks, such as Guittard

1 cup [240 ml] heavy cream

2 Tbsp Grand Marnier

1 tsp vanilla extract

½ cup [70 g] finely chopped pistachios

¼ cup [60 g] crème fraîche

Luxardo maraschino cherries in syrup

Preheat the oven to 350°F [180°C].

Combine the almond flour, cocoa powder, melted butter, maple syrup, and ¼ tsp salt in a bowl. Use a fork to mix thoroughly. Using your hands, press the dough into a 9 in [23 cm] fluted tart pan so it is flat across the bottom and comes all the way up the sides of the pan. (If necessary, butter the palms of your hands to prevent the dough from sticking to them as you press it into the tart pan.)

Place the tart pan on a baking sheet, and bake until the crust looks barely dry and set, 20 minutes. Place on a wire rack and let cool for 15 minutes.

Combine the chocolate and cream in a double boiler or in a bowl set over a pan of water on the stove. Stir over low heat until melted and smooth, about 2 minutes. Remove from the heat, and stir in the Grand Marnier, vanilla, and a pinch of salt.

CONTINUED

Pour the ganache into the cooled tart shell. Use a spatula to spread the ganache evenly. Allow to set at room temperature and serve within 4 hours, or cover and refrigerate overnight if you prefer a very dense texture. If serving the following day, allow to come to room temperature for an hour before serving.

Before serving, sprinkle some of the chopped pistachios around the rim of the tart. Dust with a little cocoa powder if desired. Garnish each slice with a spoonful of crème fraîche and a spoonful of cherries in their syrup, and sprinkle with the remaining chopped pistachios. Serve.

MATCHA PANNA COTTA

We all know matcha is taking over the planet in its tea-like form, but its cool green color and unique flavor are taking over the dessert world as well. From croissants dipped in matcha-flavored white chocolate to matcha-frosted gingerbread cookies, I think I've seen it all. I wanted to create a dessert that offered the health benefits of matcha while contrasting its earthiness with sweet ingredients. The coconut milk makes this panna cotta silky-smooth and luxurious.

When working with ground matcha, it's imperative to add a very small amount of liquid at first in order to create a smooth paste. Once that is accomplished, you can add more liquid and be guaranteed it will be lump-free. Passing the mixture through a fine-mesh strainer at the end will further ensure a smooth panna cotta.

PREPARATION TIME
15 minutes
(plus 3 hours to chill)

SERVES
6

Two 13½ oz (400 ml) cans full-fat coconut milk

2½ tsp unflavored gelatin

1 Tbsp green matcha powder, plus more for garnish

¼ cup [60 ml] light-colored maple syrup

1 tsp vanilla extract

Pinch of kosher salt

2 Tbsp black sesame seeds for garnish

8 oz [225 g] raspberries for garnish

Before opening the cans of coconut milk, shake them vigorously. This will help distribute the fat more evenly. Pour ½ cup [120 ml] of the coconut milk into a medium bowl, and sprinkle the gelatin over the top. Set aside.

Combine the matcha and 2 Tbsp of the remaining coconut milk in a small saucepan. Whisk until there are no lumps and the matcha is fully incorporated into the milk. Slowly pour in a little more of the remaining coconut milk, whisking as you go, to incorporate the matcha. Whisk in the remaining coconut milk, then add the maple syrup, vanilla, and salt. Place the saucepan over low heat. Warm until there are bubbles around the edge and it begins to steam.

CONTINUED

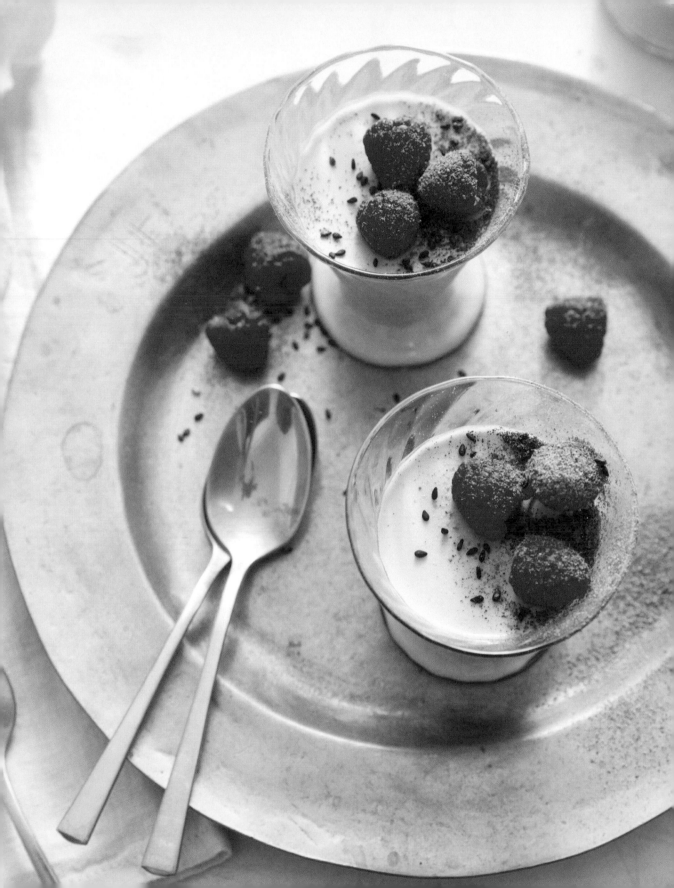

Slowly pour 2 Tbsp of the hot matcha liquid over the gelatin mixture, whisking constantly to prevent lumps and dissolve the gelatin. Continue adding the liquid, whisking the entire time. Pour the liquid through a fine-mesh strainer to remove any clumps of gelatin or matcha. Ladle the panna cotta into six small bowls or wineglasses. Cover with plastic wrap and refrigerate until set, at least 3 hours or overnight.

Just before serving, dust with a little matcha powder if desired, sprinkle a few black sesame seeds over each of the panna cotta, then top with a few raspberries. Serve.

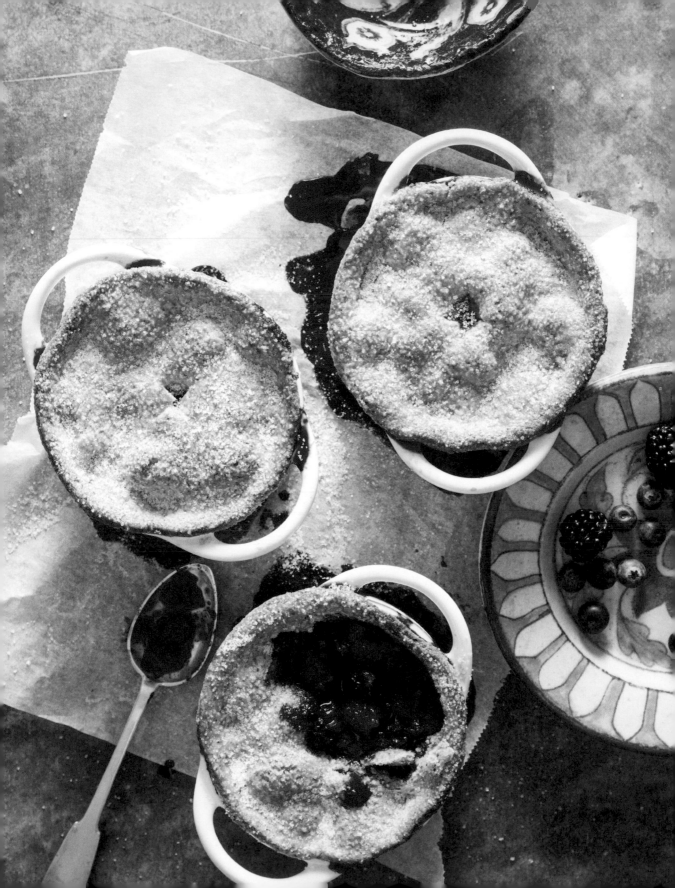

SUMMER BERRY POT PIES

This delicious recipe was a total mistake. I wanted to make a crostata, but the dough wasn't holding together as planned. (Dang gluten-free experiment!) Instead, it became more of a cookie dough, and I used a round cookie cutter to punch out pieces of dough, placed mounds of berries in ramekins, and topped each one with a slice of dough. What came out of the oven were these adorable, bubbly pot pies with a sugar cookie–like crust. For fun, use other shapes of cookie cutters for the dough, like stars or hearts.

You'll need twelve 6 oz [180 ml] ramekins for this recipe. If you don't own them, you can purchase disposable aluminum ones.

PREPARATION TIME

30 minutes
(plus 1 hour to chill the dough)

COOKING TIME
25 minutes
(plus 20 minutes to cool)

SERVES
12

CRUST

1½ cups [240 g] gluten-free flour, such as Cup4Cup or Bob's Red Mill	1 tsp kosher salt
1 cup [110 g] almond flour	¾ cup [165 g] unsalted butter, cold, cut into 10 pieces
⅓ cup [100 g] sugar, plus more for sprinkling	2 eggs plus 1 egg yolk

BERRY FILLING

2 lb [910 g] strawberries, hulled and quartered	1 cup [200 g] sugar
12 oz [340 g] blueberries	2 Tbsp cornstarch
12 oz [340 g] raspberries	1 Tbsp grated lemon zest
12 oz [340 g] blackberries	2 tsp vanilla extract
	1 tsp kosher salt

CONTINUED

To make the crust: In the bowl of a food processor fitted with a metal blade, combine the flours, sugar, and salt. Pulse to combine. Add the butter and pulse until the mixture resembles coarse sand. Add 1 egg and the egg yolk, and continue to pulse until the dough comes together and begins to form a ball. If the dough seems too dry and does not stick together when lightly squeezed, add up to 1 Tbsp water and pulse to combine. Turn the dough out onto a clean work surface dusted with flour. Work the dough into a ball and then flatten into a disk about 2 in [5 cm] thick. The dough will be slightly crumbly. Wrap the disk tightly in plastic and refrigerate for 1 hour.

To make the berry filling: Combine all the ingredients in a large bowl. Let stand at room temperature until ready to use. Transfer ¾ cup [180 g] of the filling to a 6 oz [180 g] ramekin, making sure the filling goes to the top. Repeat with the remaining ramekins, and place on a baking sheet.

Preheat the oven to 350°F [180°C]. Generously flour a clean work surface and roll out the dough with a floured rolling pin to ¼ in [6 mm] thickness. Using a 3½ in [9 cm] round cookie cutter or drinking glass, cut out 12 rounds. Use a small offset spatula or knife to transfer the dough rounds to the ramekins, placing them on top of the berries and pressing down slightly. Whisk the remaining egg in a small bowl, then brush the dough lightly with the egg and sprinkle with sugar.

Bake until the crusts are cooked through and slightly golden, about 25 minutes. Set aside to cool for 20 minutes, then serve.

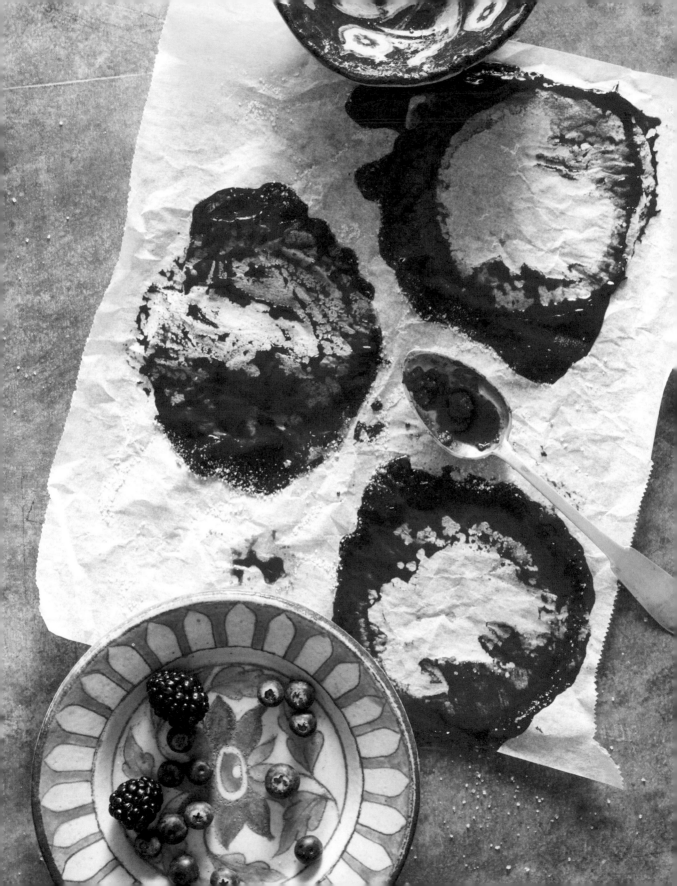

ORANGE-TARRAGON GRANITA

I'm tarragon-obsessed and always looking for new ways to use it. So, when I was brainstorming this granita, Inken Chrisman, one of my amazing recipe developers, suggested trying it in place of mint. It's spectacular! This granita would be perfect on a really hot day after a barbecue, or equally as good served after a lighter luncheon with salad and grilled shrimp. And if you can't find tarragon, of course you can use mint.

PREPARATION TIME
20 minutes (plus 2 hours to freeze)

SERVES
4–6

⅓ cup [65 g] sugar

⅓ cup [80 ml] water

4 sprigs fresh tarragon plus ¼ cup [8 g] chopped fresh tarragon

3 cups [720 ml] fresh orange juice

2 Tbsp fresh lemon juice

In a small saucepan over medium-high heat, combine the sugar, water, and tarragon sprigs. Bring to a simmer, stirring to dissolve the sugar. Let cool for about 15 minutes. Strain the tarragon simple syrup through a fine-mesh sieve into a clean container.

In a large bowl, stir together the orange juice, lemon juice, and tarragon simple syrup. Pour into a 9 by 13 in [23 by 33 cm] baking pan. Transfer to the freezer for 30 minutes. Stir with a fork, scraping up the icy parts. Return to the freezer, scraping with a fork every 30 minutes, until the mixture is frozen and has the texture of shaved ice, about 2 hours total.

Sprinkle with the chopped tarragon, and use a fork to evenly distribute. Serve immediately.

See photo on page 176.

TEQUILA OLD-FASHIONEDS
with Luxardo Cherries

When I entertain, cocktails are typically involved—and I especially love tequila. So when I got to know the lovely Casamigos cocktail brand, I followed them on Instagram. Their hashtag is #houseoffriends. Never one to shy away from a good pun, I started tagging my tequila pics with #haasoffriends. Rande Gerber, one of the founders, was kind enough to send me their tequila book with my hashtag written in it next to theirs! Casamigos and I are now married.

With this cocktail, I wanted to do justice to their reposado, a tequila that has been aged in whiskey barrels for seven months. It's delicious on its own, but for those of you who are new to sipping tequila, I wanted to add another layer of flavor. Enter the Luxardo cherries and lime juice. I freeze the cherries in 1 in [2.5 cm] square ice cube trays in some cherry juice, and finish each drink with a splash of lime juice to balance the sweetness. Drink this and feel like a total grown-up.

PREPARATION TIME
10 minutes (plus 4 hours to freeze the ice cubes)

SERVES
6

12 Luxardo maraschino cherries, plus 4 Tbsp [60 ml] of their syrup

1½ cups [360 ml] cherry juice

9 oz [270 ml] reposado tequila

2 Tbsp fresh lime juice

To make the ice cubes, place a cherry and 1 tsp of its syrup in the bottom of each mold of an ice cube tray. Fill the molds with cherry juice. Freeze until the ice cubes are firm, at least 4 hours.

When ready to serve the cocktails, place 2 ice cubes in each double old-fashioned glass. Pour 1½ oz [45 ml] of reposado over the ice cubes, then top with 1 tsp lime juice. Serve immediately.

HERB GARDEN GIN *and* TONIC

I pride myself on tending an awesome bar, as I think my true calling is entertaining people and making sure their plates are full and they are never without a good drink! But in the context of aging well, excessive alcohol has no place, so I wanted to create cocktails that were absolutely delicious with a redeeming quality or two! I wouldn't call this gin and tonic health food, but it is so full of beautiful herbs and flowers I'm convinced it might be a little bit good for us.

PREPARATION TIME
5 minutes

SERVES
1

4 oz [120 ml] Fever-Tree tonic	Dried lavender
2 oz [60 ml] St. George gin	Lime, for garnish
2 dashes Angostura bitters	Fennel fronds, violets, and/or fresh herbs, such as flowering basil, bay leaf, parsley, rosemary, and/or dill, for garnish
Fennel pollen	

Fill a rocks glass with ice. Add the tonic, gin, and bitters. Stir to combine. Sprinkle with fennel pollen and dried lavender. Top with lime and fresh herbs, add a fennel frond and some violets, and serve.

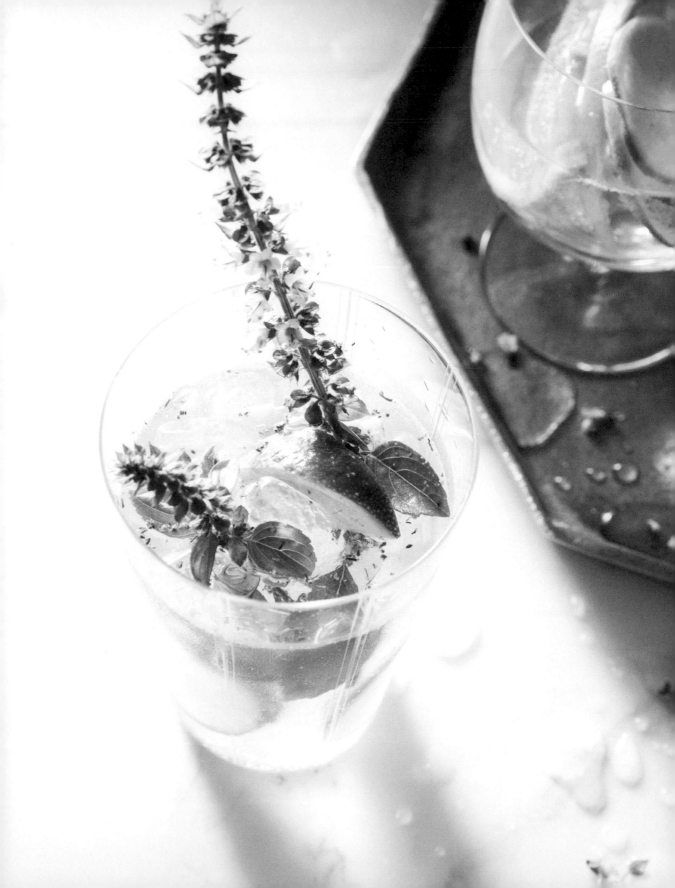

SAUVIGNON BLANC SANGRIA

To me, sangria screams "party!" It's loaded with gorgeous ingredients, you can make it in batches before you entertain, and there is something for everyone in it! Instead of the traditional combo of apples and oranges—frankly, not my favorite—I use raspberries and grapefruit, a combo I love!

PREPARATION TIME
5 minutes
(plus 2 hours to chill)

SERVES
8

⅓ cup [65 g] sugar

⅓ cup [80 ml] water

1 [750-ml] bottle dry, fruity Sauvignon Blanc

4 oz [120 ml] Grand Marnier

4 oz [115 g] raspberries

1 lime, thinly sliced

½ grapefruit, thinly sliced

2 cups [480 ml] sparkling water

In a small saucepan over medium-high heat, combine the sugar and water. Bring to a simmer, stirring to dissolve the sugar. Let cool for about 15 minutes.

In a tall pitcher, stir together the Sauvignon Blanc, Grand Marnier, and ¼ cup [60 ml] of the simple syrup (discard the remainder). Add the raspberries, lime, and grapefruit. Refrigerate for at least 2 hours or up to 6 hours. Just before serving, add the sparkling water and stir gently.

AMANDA'S CALIFORNIA COCKTAIL

I am obsessed with St-Germain, the elderflower liqueur that takes everything from basic to delightful in one sip. It pairs so nicely with floral gins and vodkas. I love to use it when friends tell me they only like vodka, but want something a little different. A splash of this in your vodka cocktail along with some citrus feels like what the rest of the world imagines life to be like in California—light, sunny, and happy!

   If you prefer to serve this up, it would be delicious shaken and served in a martini glass without the added soda water or garnishes.

PREPARATION TIME
5 minutes

SERVES
1

1½ oz [45 ml] high-quality vodka, such as Blue Ice, Tito's, or Grey Goose

½ oz [15 ml] St-Germain liqueur

1 slice of grapefruit plus 1 Tbsp fresh grapefruit juice

Soda water

1 sprig rosemary

Combine the vodka, St. Germain, and grapefruit juice in a cocktail shaker. Add ice and shake. Strain into a glass that has ice cubes in it. Add the slice of grapefruit so it's sitting vertically in the glass. Top with soda water and garnish with a rosemary sprig. Serve.

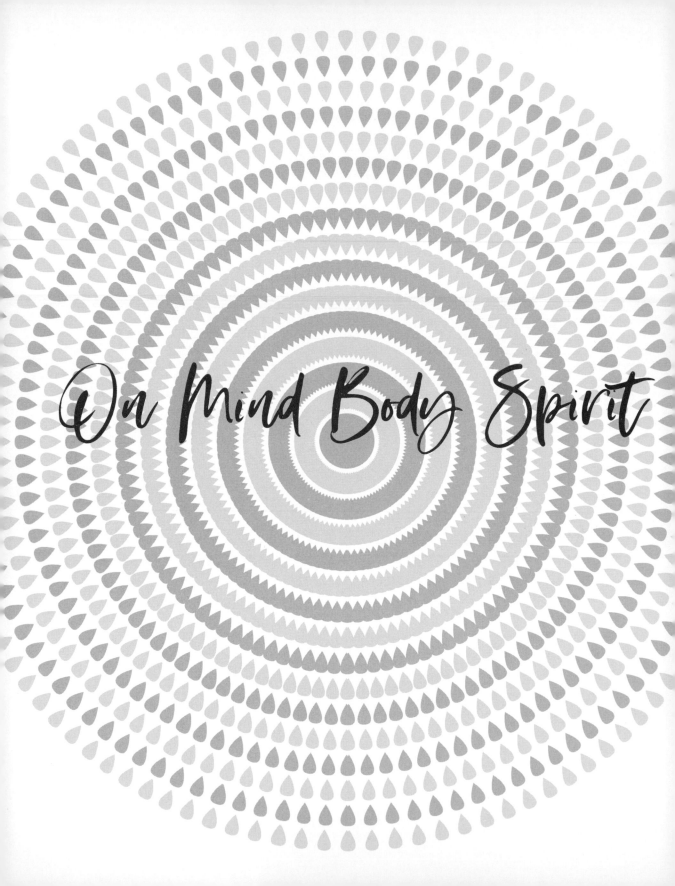

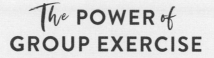

The POWER of GROUP EXERCISE

with SoulCycle coaches Stephanie Peters
and Sumner Weldon

When it comes to exercise, I've always been a bit of a loner. In a class setting I can get easily intimidated by the people who seem to know all the moves. Also, I injured my back thirty years ago and to this day, I feel embarrassed when I have to adapt the movements to work for me.

But as I started to write this book, I realized my body needed more exercise than I was giving it, and when left to my own devices, I naturally forfeit exercise whenever it competes with coffee, meditation, or my eight hours of sleep.

Some friends had been encouraging me to try a class at SoulCycle for ages. At first, I was afraid I would be terrible at it. I'd heard it was impossibly difficult and not for the faint of heart. Finally, a friend convinced me to tag along. The first time I went, I picked a spot in the very back. The room was pretty dark, which I loved, because it allowed me to be in my thoughts and focus on my own work instead of comparing myself to others in the class.

As the teacher started talking to us, she shared so many motivational thoughts, reminding us that we are in control of our actions, our bodies, and how great—or awful—our lives can be, and that simply showing up to work on ourselves for forty-five minutes that morning was an indicator that we can make positive choices every day. In addition to feeling uplifted and motivated, I found myself trying much harder than I would have if I were cycling by myself. Time flew by as I was singing along to my favorite song one moment, quietly in my thoughts at another, and remembering what it felt like to really push myself, something I hadn't done physically in a long time. (Strangely enough, I found myself crying a lot, because I could finally quiet my mind enough to think about what changes I needed to make in my life.)

I walked out of there as red as a tomato, but I was hooked. What was it that made that experience so unique? As I went back time and time again, I realized one thing: the instructors were creating an atmosphere that was charged with positive energy, and it was palpable.

In addition to getting a boost of endorphins—which help us sleep better and feel less stressed, and act as a natural painkiller—I was walking out of that room feeling truly boosted by the people around me. I was so encouraged by everyone in the room trying their hardest to excel, and cheering each other on.

Which led me to ask myself another question: was the collective group creating an energy that I couldn't create by myself?

I had a sense that it was, but I wanted to know more. I started by asking my two favorite SoulCycle instructors, Stephanie Peters and Sumner Weldon, a few questions about the power of group energy.

Amanda Haas: What do you think is so special about cycling as a group versus doing it alone?

Stephanie Peters: Working out in a group fitness setting makes it fun and much more motivating! For years, I used to go to the gym by myself and I never liked it. It was a case of checking it off my list. Once I started attending, and then later teaching, classes at SoulCycle, I always looked forward to going because the energy of the room lifts you up and makes the workout go by faster. You also meet amazing people! The SoulCycle community in particular is very strong. I've met some of my best friends in these classes, and that's something that never happened when I worked out alone.

Sumner Weldon: There's something so special about being in a dark, candlelit room with fifty-five other people. You feel and feed off each other's infectious energy and positive vibes. Together we create forty-five minutes of pushing each other out of our comfort zones. Being surrounded by other riders helps provide not only the support you need to discover what you can accomplish inside the room, but also a confidence that you can take out into the world and apply to everyday life. How you do one thing is how you do everything. I truly believe that "your vibe attracts your tribe." So it's important to surround yourself (even in a workout) with people who will lift you up while taking your life (or fitness) to the next level.

AH: How does group energy motivate people differently than an individual alone?

SP: The group energy makes it easier to work out and much more enjoyable. You have the instructor and all of the other riders encouraging you. The adrenaline is pumping through every person in the room. You can feel that positive energy, and it helps carry you through the class and push yourself harder than you would otherwise. When you work out alone, you have to do all of the motivating yourself, which can make it really difficult to stay consistent.

SW: Let's be honest, we all wake up and have days where we're in a funky mood or too tired to get through a workout alone in the living room or garage. Sometimes you just need the motivation of someone leading you or pushing through.

AH: What do you set out to do for people in each class?

SP: First and foremost, I set out to give people the best physical workout possible. I also really try to make the class fun so that it goes by quickly and people look forward to coming. Just because it's exercise doesn't mean it has to be torture! It is also important to me to create a safe environment where riders do not have to worry about being perfect. I want them to be motivated to do their best, whatever that is on that particular day, without feeling pressure to get all the moves right!

SW: I provide a service to my riders each and every day. I take a few minutes to clear my head so that I can be present and relatable with my message every class.

AH: How do you continue to stay motivated to exercise like you do?

SP: The key for me is that I always feel amazing after a workout. I have never left one thinking, "I wish I had just stayed home on the couch and watched TV." I also really look forward to seeing the same people in the classes that I teach and attend. Working out with them every day inspires me to teach the best possible class and to push myself harder.

SW: Being an instructor at SoulCycle is literally my dream job. Previously, I was a professional dancer in LA, so movement and music are my passion. Put them both together and you see this energetic, passionate person who can't stop smiling or dancing around the room. When you love what you do, it doesn't feel like a job.

After talking with Stephanie and Sumner, I had answered my question about group exercise with an unequivocal "YES!" in my mind, but I still wanted a little more proof to back me up. I turned to the book *Subtle Energy: Awakening to the Unseen Forces in Our Lives* by William Collinge, Ph.D., which details fascinating discoveries made at the HeartMath Institute in Boulder Creek, California. One such study examined whether heart energy could be transferred from person to person when subjects were 3 ft [1 m] apart, not touching, and wired with electrodes. The electrocardiogram in the experiment detected energy across the space between the people on the surface of each other's bodies. This shows that heart energy can be radiated between people in close proximity—even when they aren't touching.

Aha!

Whether it's because of the energy of others that is lifting me up, or something as scientific as our hearts' electromagnetic fields extending throughout a room, I've fallen in love with group exercise. And now, I've gained the confidence to be in the front row, not because I've mastered the moves, but because I thrive on the positive energy I'm absorbing through Steph, Sumner, and the other riders around me.

LOVE *the* SKIN YOU'RE IN

with dermatologist Kelly Hood

As I've aged, I've had few regrets. But I do regret living a sunscreen-free life in Arizona for twenty-two years. My summers as a kid consisted of contests to get the best tan lines possible, which meant zero sunscreen and, even worse, putting baby oil on my skin after swim team practice to speed things up! Luckily, I started seeing a dermatologist in high school and he was able to treat the areas of my skin that had already formed precancerous cells due to overexposure to the sun.

By the time I moved to San Francisco at twenty-two, I'd gotten the message: use sunscreen and keep your skin protected if you want to age well! I went from being a sun worshiper to basically staying covered at all times and spending very little time at the beach. My skin thanked me for it, but there was no reversing some of my sun damage, like the freckles on my lips, which are a telltale sign of too much sun.

As the world of injectables has grown exponentially, many people associate dermatologists with beauty or vanity—the place people go to get a little dose of Botox or other filler to turn back the clock. But having a dermatologist in your life to take care of your skin—your body's largest organ—is vital to good health. I make sure to visit Dr. Kelly Hood annually, so she can check my skin for anything unusual.

A bit about Dr. Hood: She is a board-certified dermatologist in Lafayette, California. She's a spokesperson for the American Academy of Dermatology and a member of the American Society of Dermatologic Surgeons, the San Francisco Dermatologic Society, and California Cosmetic Dermatologists. Basically, she is awesome.

One thing I appreciate about Dr. Hood is that she's honest with patients about what fillers can do for them. Since I spend a lot of time in front of a camera, she recommended I stay away from them; she doesn't want me to look fake. (That didn't stop me from asking her to do a little on my forehead and around my eyes. The verdict? I loved that the wrinkles in my forehead had diminished, but when I looked at pictures of myself, I could tell that areas of my face no longer matched.)

My take on my aging skin: it's not about reversing the clock. I want to look my age, but a great version of myself for my age. Dr. Hood has been wonderful in helping me achieve this, so I sat down to ask her some of the questions we all want to know about aging skin. Here she is in her own words.

DR. KELLY HOOD:

Aging is associated with changes in the skin, which generally come from declining repair mechanisms. Some skin changes are genetic and related to ethnicity. In general, in our twenties, our natural antioxidants begin to decrease. In our thirties, a decrease in sun-damage repair mechanisms occurs. Our skin in our forties shows progressive senescence, or biological aging. In our fifth decade, the skin barrier building blocks begin to malfunction. As the skin barrier malfunctions, our skin becomes dry and cracked. These changes occur in both sun-exposed and sun-protected areas but are exacerbated in sun-damaged skin. As our population ages, much research is devoted to understanding and treating or preventing these alterations.

We wear our skin for our entire lives. The main goal of the cosmeceutical industry is to prevent or reverse skin changes that occur over our lifetime. The most important products to date for naturally taking care of the skin are sunscreens, moisturizers, retinoids, and antioxidants. Sun protection is the number one most important thing. One can appreciate this by comparing the skin of the face and arms to the sun-protected skin of the buttocks. Elastosis (loss of elasticity) of the skin causes that crinkly look in sun-exposed areas.

Skin aging results from extrinsic and intrinsic aging. Photoaging is premature skin aging accelerated by sun exposure. Intrinsic aging is the natural aging that occurs in all cells. Chronic damage from the sun's ultraviolet light results in most of the age-associated changes in the appearance of skin, such as skin thinning, blotchiness, lines, redness, and skin cancer.

SUN EXPOSURE

The sun gives us daylight and vitamin D, but it is also detrimental to the beauty of our skin if we're overexposed. Sunscreens do not prevent sunburn or tanning; they prolong the time we can spend in the sun before tanning and burning occur. Sunscreens that protect against ultraviolet B (short waves, or UVB) and ultraviolet A (long waves, or UVA) should be applied to the face and neck every day. UVB sunscreens protect against overexposure from the sun-burning rays that cause DNA damage. UVA protection provides defense against UVA wavelengths produced by the sun and emitted by light bulbs. UVA wavelengths tend to penetrate deep into the epidermis and dermis, causing pigment disruption and skin thinning mainly through

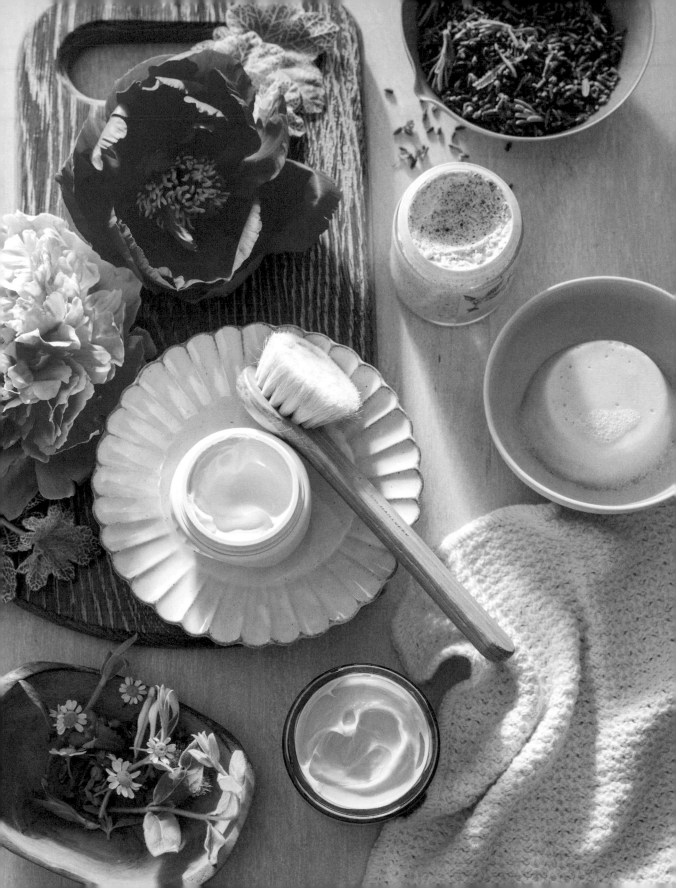

production of free radicals (oxidative stress). For your daily sunscreen, I recommend at least SPF 30 UVA/UVB sunscreen, which blocks out approximately 7 percent of UV radiation.

Sunscreen can prevent sun damage if applied properly. An ounce of sunscreen—enough to fill a shot glass—applied to your exposed skin is generally considered the amount needed for prolonged sun protection. Remember that no sunscreen is "waterproof." If you're perspiring or in the water, quick reapplication is necessary. Of course, sunscreen is no substitute for sun avoidance and protective clothing.

Sunburn can be immediately temporized with aspirin or ibuprofen and N-acetyl cysteine. This reduces "sunburn cells," which cause inflammation and pain. Anti-inflammatories such as aspirin and ibuprofen actually decrease DNA damage to skin cells.

If you've already had too much sun exposure, there are still some ways to reverse the effects. Remember that the skin is constantly regenerating, so protecting the skin from damaging sunrays will result in a cosmetic improvement of the skin. Retinoids and antioxidants can help prevent and reverse sun damage as well. However, avoiding sun damage is much easier than reversing sun damage.

BEST PRODUCTS FOR SKIN CARE

Topical retinoids have the potential to address sun-damaged skin. Retinoids neutralize some of the damage caused by the sun and can actually prevent or reverse some symptoms of skin aging, such as clumping of pigment, which cause brown spots, and thinning of the skin, which can cause crepiness and dryness. The FDA-approved, scientifically substantiated products are tretinoin (Retin A) and tazarotene (Tazorac). It generally takes three to six months of daily use to see significant improvement. Smoother skin, a rosy glow, decrease in blotchy pigmentation, and diminished fine lines and wrinkles occur over time.

Topical antioxidants are meant to protect against and reverse damage caused by the environment. The advantage of applying antioxidants rather than ingesting them is that the skin attains a higher concentration and the skin maintains a reservoir of antioxidant that cannot be rubbed or washed off for several days. Oxygen is necessary for our survival but is also associated with our aging. An oxygen environment generates free radicals, which in turn cause oxidation. Oxidation causes degeneration, as seen in rusted metal. Oxidation of the skin causes changes associated with aging, such as dark spots, wrinkles, and thinning.

The most-studied antioxidants used for skin enhancement are vitamin C and vitamin E. There is great variation in products available, but check the ingredients—when you see vitamin C or E toward the end of an ingredient list, it means it's probably not present in a large enough amount to do much.

Moisturizers are important for the appearance of skin. As we age, our cells do not retain water as well, which gives the skin a dull, lusterless appearance. Moisturizers hold water in the cells and reduce water evaporation. My favorite inexpensive moisturizer is sunflower oil. It is the oil most closely related to our natural skin oils.

THE FOODS YOU EAT

Many patients ask me if certain foods can make their skin look better or worse. In general, fruits and vegetables maintain and can improve skin health. Adequate amounts of vitamins C, E, and A are an absolute requirement. Whether skin vitamin supplements are effective is not proven. There is no substitute for a balanced and varied healthy diet based on non-processed foods. Good foods help prevent inflammation, which can lead to type 2 diabetes, cancer (including skin cancer), and neurodegenerative diseases, all of which affect health and appearance. Sugar is the main culprit in many skin health disorders, including acne, itching, eczema, and psoriasis. The severity of acne can be directly correlated to sugar intake. Gluten sensitivity can also cause acne and rashes.

THE TAKEAWAY

When it comes to skin care, the best thing to remember is that the way we treat our body is reflected in our skin. Eat a healthy diet heavy on the vegetables and fruits. Avoid fast food, cigarettes, and excessive sun exposure. Get plenty of rest and aerobic exercise. Wear moisturizing sunscreen every day on your face, neck, and exposed chest. I like a two-in-one moisturizing sunscreen—it makes application quick and easy. Antioxidants and retinoids are important to reverse skin damage and protect against further insult. Control your stress. Remember not to become overzealous with cosmetic procedures. If one has too much done, one looks "done." Self-care and confidence go a long way.

MEDITATION *for* SELF-LOVE

with meditation teacher and practitioner Hailey Lott

Over the past decade, I've made some room in my life for meditation. I took a few classes, spent five to twenty minutes a day (when I remembered) trying to practice, and noticed small changes. But as I really examined my health for this book and spent time recovering from surgery on my parathyroid gland, person after person kept urging me to make meditation a real and regular part of my life.

Hailey Lott has had a deep impact on the growth of my meditation practice. Just out of college but already a practiced meditator when I met her, Hailey immediately blew me away, reminding me once again that age is simply a number. You don't have to be eighty-five to have wisdom or be spiritually grounded. Hailey has practiced and studied meditation for fifteen years. She studied under Brother Phap Sieu, who personally studied under Thich Naht Hanh, to take her practice to the next level and become a teacher.

I invited Hailey to share her thoughts on meditation and offer four guided meditations themed around self-love and inner calm. Here's what she had to say.

HAILEY LOTT:

If you have meditated before—even just a little—but still aren't experiencing the life-changing, mind-pausing benefits, then these practices will be your answer. If you're feeling a little lost and wondering how something as simple as meditation can impact your life, keep reading.

I began meditating over fifteen years ago when my mother, God bless her, asked our family to sit around the dinner table and meditate together (this would sound woo-woo to most but was somewhat normal for us since we grew up doing family yoga and drinking crystal-infused water!). My-ten-year-old self closed her eyes and her thoughts got louder, her patience got smaller, and her ability to sit still was completely nonexistent. I could not handle the pressure of being with just me and my thoughts. Maybe you've sat in meditation and similarly felt your thoughts getting louder, as if you opened up the cage of a Tasmanian devil. If this is you, welcome to the club.

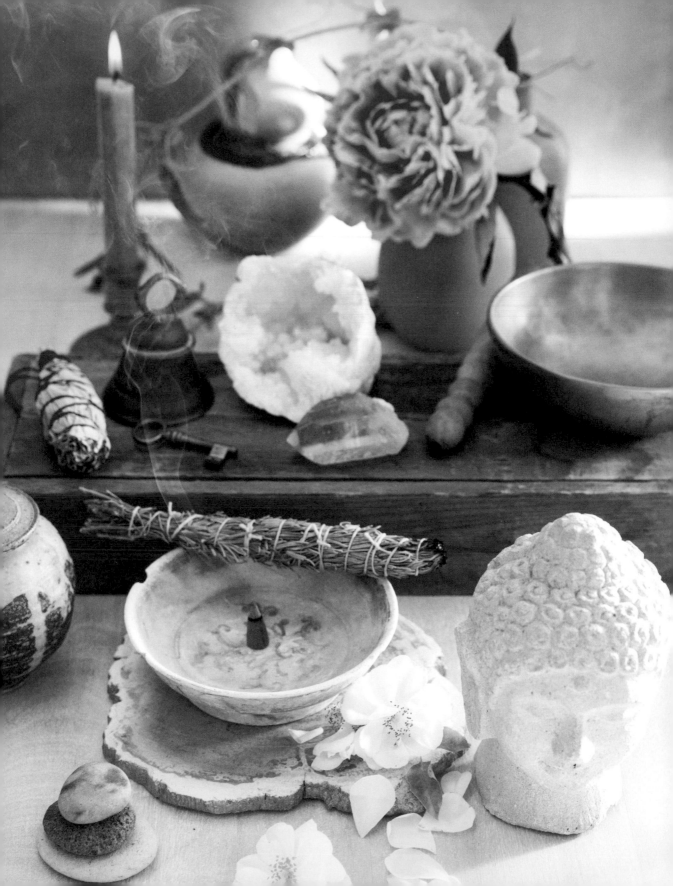

One thing to remember is that you are just beginning. This is a time to give your-self compassion, love, and acceptance for being where you are. Wherever you are in this practice is absolutely perfect. And in fact, if you aren't yet your own biggest cheerleader, then get ready to start practicing some self-love.

World-renowned meditation teacher, bestselling author, and one of my per-sonal role models, Sharon Salzberg, writes, "Meditation is essentially training our attention so that we can be more aware—not only of our own inner workings but also of what's happening around us in the here and now." In meditation, you practice becoming the observer of your thoughts. You begin to see your thoughts, stories, and judgments for what they truly are: neutral. Alarms may be going off for you right now. You may be saying to yourself, "But how can being diagnosed with a serious health condition—or being hurt by this person or that situation—be neutral?" My answer to you is that whatever you say it is, it will be. You can choose to look at the health diagnosis as the end of your life or as the beginning of your health journey toward discovering techniques to heal from the inside out. You can look at the argu-ment you just had with your friend or partner as devastating or you can step back and see it as an opportunity for growth—possibly even a chance to be vulnerable and honest with this person and deepen the relationship with mutual understanding. We are meaning-making machines, most often operating in overdrive, creating false realities around everything from the parking ticket we got to the way one of our coworkers glanced at us funny.

Does that mind-set serve you? We have the power to create our own reality and experience by what we choose to notice and by the meaning we give each situation or circumstance. And once you know that you are in control of your own reality, wouldn't you want to put a positive spin on it? This is exactly what we practice as we sit in meditation. We take a back seat to the thoughts that rule our mind and simply notice that they are there. We stop attaching to them and start letting them go.

A pivotal study on meditation done by the neuroscientist Sara Lazar of Harvard in 2005 gives us some insight into how meditation affects the brain. This study, made up of ordinary Boston-area professionals, most of whom meditated for around forty minutes a day, showed that regular practitioners of meditation had measurably thicker tissue in the left prefrontal cortex of the brain, the area responsible for cog-nitive and emotional processing and well-being. What's even more fascinating is what researchers saw in the brain scans of the older participants in the study. The scans showed that meditation can actually *reverse* the thinning of the cortex that occurs naturally with aging. This means that meditation can protect against many of the things that typically happen to an aging brain, including memory loss and decreased focus. So yeah, this meditation thing really works!

I've created four meditations you can do at home (or anywhere!). Each is designed to support you in a different way with the ultimate goals of self-love and inner calm. I recommend trying them all at first and then using each as needed in different moments and situations throughout your day.

SETTLING INTO MEDITATION

To set yourself up for a successful meditation, find a quiet space where you can sit undisturbed. To make this space extra-special, place in it your favorite scented candle, a treasured trinket, or anything that makes you feel warm, comforted, and relaxed. The goal is to create a sacred space for you to just be. Each meditation is designed to be around ten minutes long, so if setting a timer is your thing, go for it! If not, just pay attention to what feels good in your body; it will tell you when the meditation is complete.

Ideally you will sit up straight on a pillow or maybe in a chair. Lying down is great as long as you aren't extremely tired—we don't want you to fall asleep and miss all the good stuff! When you've settled into a comfortable seated position, place the meditation in front of you to read out loud. Because some of the meditations are long, I suggest reading them once and recording yourself on your phone (be sure to speak slowly and calmly in a soothing voice), and then playing back the recording while you sit. This will help you transition into your meditation and support you in feeling the words in every cell in your body. While playing the meditation, you can choose to keep your eyes open and focus on one specific point, or keep your eyes closed.

As you begin to meditate, turn inward and focus awareness on your breath. Notice what your breath feels like in your body. Bring your awareness to any areas of tension or tightness in your body and send your breath there to ease those muscles. Continue to let go and come into a deeper state of relaxation. As you sit, practice seeing any thoughts that come up. Notice the thoughts and simply let them go. You may do this a hundred times in just one minute and that's OK! Continue to practice and the thoughts will become quieter and your mind will let go more quickly. There isn't a right or wrong, good or bad, way to meditate. Let the process be explorative.

As you move into your practice, I ask you to commit to sit in meditation every day for thirty days, even if it's just for five minutes. So tomorrow set your alarm for five minutes earlier, hop out of bed, and sit—it's that easy! We all deserve a few minutes for ourselves.

MEDITATION 1: LETTING GO

This meditation is designed to support you in letting go of your anxieties and worries. It will bring you back to your peaceful and neutral home base. Use this practice when you feel like screaming but you can't because you're at the office, working the school bake sale, or anywhere in public.

Bring all of your attention and focus to the breath. Use the power of your breath to bring you in to this present moment. As you feel the breath in the body, begin to count each breath as it enters and exits your body.

Breathe in (one).

Breathe out (two).

In (three).

Out (four).

Repeat this up to the number ten and then start over.

If you lose focus, gently redirect your mind back to counting your breath and begin again at one. When you are ready, you can gently let go of the counting and begin to bring the words *calm* and *ease* to your mind.

As you inhale, silently repeat the word *calm*. As you exhale, silently repeat the word *ease*. Feel these words travel throughout your entire body. Allow the words to take over your mind. What does it feel like to create calm and ease throughout the mind and the body?

Remember this calm and ease throughout the rest of your day and tap back into this feeling simply by focusing on the breath.

Begin to deepen the breath.

On this next breath, hold at the top . . . and let all the air go.

When you are ready, you can wiggle your fingers and toes. Tap back in to all of your senses. Gently flutter open your eyes.

MEDITATION 2: BODY LOVE

This practice was created to support you in finding the beautiful, unique, and divine state that your body is in right now. Our reality begins in our mind, so practice shifting your thoughts from self-deprecating to self-accepting and watch as your body fills with self-love.

Bring all of your attention and focus to the breath. Use the power of your breath to bring you in to this present moment.

Begin to bring to mind different parts of your body. Going from head to toe, show deep appreciation for each body part and what it provides for you. As each body part comes to mind, express gratitude for that area. Thank your feet for grounding you, your legs for carrying you, your stomach for its intuition and guidance, your mouth for nourishing you.

Now I invite you to bring to mind your body in its ideal shape. Notice what your arms feel like, your legs. Begin to notice how your whole body feels. What is the expression on your face? What are you doing with your body in its ideal shape? What does it feel like for you to love your body so deeply?

Acknowledge that you've nourished your body with good food and taken care of your body with rest. Honor your body for everything it has overcome. Know that your healthiest shape is something you always have access to when you cherish your body, love your body, and accept your body as it is in this moment.

Now invite into your mind's eye a word or phrase of appreciation for your body. As you form this mantra, begin to silently repeat the word or phrase in your mind. Continue the repetition, filling up your body with kindness, compassion, and love. Imagine placing this word or phrase over your heart. Reach for it whenever you want to appreciate your beautiful body and everything it has done for you.

Slowly begin to deepen the breath, and notice the rise and fall of your belly. Begin to wiggle your fingers and toes, and slowly open your eyes.

MEDITATION 3: IDEAL SELF

This meditation is designed to support you in seeing your greatness, your charm, and all the gifts you have to offer the world. It is designed to fill you up with inspiration and healing so that you can go through your day with confidence and ease.

Bring all of your attention and focus to the breath. Use the power of your breath to bring you in to this present moment. As you turn your energy inward, see yourself letting go of any thoughts of the past and of the future.

Bring your attention to the area right behind your eyes. Allow your entire face to just soften, your shoulders to drop. Find yourself becoming the observer of your own breath.

Imagine the sun in your mind's eye. Allow everything else to dissolve. Feel the warm light of the sun cascading its rays over you. It lights up your forehead and warms your mind, comes down through your throat, your shoulders, your arms. Feel the warm light coming in through your heart, through your ribs, into your torso, into your hips.

Imagine yourself standing strong; feel the strength in your legs, your feet. Now imagine living your most ideal life. See yourself: what you are doing, who you are with, the look on your face.

You are exactly where you are meant to be.

You feel self-assured, confident, unstoppable. Think about what living your vision feels like.

Allow this feeling to spread throughout your body. Focus on what feels good and what is possible when you live your vision. Feel more confident, more self-assured with each and every breath.

Take one last deep breath in, holding it at the top, and let it all out. Slowly begin to wiggle your fingers and your toes. Rub your palms together to create a little bit of heat, and then place your palms on top of your eyes; lower your hands and gently flutter the eyes open, coming back into the room.

MEDITATION 4: CALM WITHIN A STORM

This practice was created to support you to move through anything that is thrown at you, whether you're having a particularly crazy day or you feel stuck in a stressful situation. In this meditation, you will find peace and strength and the inner knowledge that you can flow through life no matter what circumstances arise.

Settle in and slow down your breath. I invite you to bring to mind the shape of you in this meditation.

Whether you are seated or lying down, begin to picture what you look like in your mind's eye. Notice how still you are, how grounded you feel. You are unwavering. As you continue to hold this image of yourself in your mind, begin to let in whatever thoughts naturally come. See your thoughts, to-do lists, worries, and any challenge you're experiencing in this moment begin to float around this image you have of yourself in your mind's eye. See the thoughts, stories, and judgments get bigger, louder. Watch as they swirl all around you.

See the image and outline of you still strong, grounded, and unwavering. No matter what comes to you, you have the choice to stay in this space of peace and calm. Allow yourself to be the witness of your surroundings and know that your power, your strength, and your stillness all come from within. Gently let the external distractions disappear and hold on to this image of you in your power, strength, and unwavering stillness.

This is who you are and who you will always be.

Slowly bring your awareness to your body, and feel the breath get longer and deeper.

Invite in small movement to your fingers and toes. When you are ready, gently open your eyes.

SLEEP *for* YOUR HEALTH

As we humans have become more connected via technology and mobile devices, the lines between work, play, and rest have blurred. Many people I know check email and social media compulsively up until bedtime and have stopped the wonderful practice of winding down before they go to sleep. It feels like a lot of people in today's busy society view sleep as a luxury rather than a necessity. But I completely disagree. I have always loved sleep, and recognized at a very young age that I don't function well without it. (Am I the only one whose brain feels fuzzy and who can't concentrate if I've had less than seven hours?)

Because I'm such a fan of a good night's sleep—and a huge believer in naps as well—I love asking people how much sleep they think they need. My favorite responses lately have come from two successful business executives. I admire both of these women so much and have always wondered how they do it. One of them said to me, "I don't have time for sleep" and the other one answered, "I'll sleep when I'm dead." It's interesting to note they both live on caffeine, drinking it well into the afternoon. Although I admire their desire to succeed and achieve, Mother Nature dictates that sleep is absolutely imperative for good health and for high-level functioning. And you can't argue with Mother Nature!

When researching sleep for this book, I simply wanted to study the benefits of good sleep on our bodies, and what happens when we continually deprive ourselves of sleep. Luckily, the National Institutes of Health (NIH) has doctors devoted solely to sleep research.

SO WHAT ARE THE BENEFITS OF GETTING GOOD SLEEP?

According to Merrill Mitler, a sleep expert and neuroscientist at the NIH, a good night's sleep is fundamental to learning, memory, and clear thinking, and to hold good focus. In addition, high-quality sleep can help us react more quickly, keeping our reflexes sharp. Michael Twery, another sleep expert at NIH, also shared that sleep affects every tissue in our bodies. It can affect growth and stress hormones, improve our immunity, curb inflammation, reduce blood pressure, enhance our moods, and help us maintain a healthy weight.

WHAT HAPPENS IF WE DON'T GET GOOD SLEEP?

A loss of sleep can impair our ability to reason, solve problems, and pay attention to detail. It can also affect our moods, making us more susceptible to depression. Studies find a lack of sleep to be associated with many diseases, including diabetes, heart disease, stroke, and kidney disease, to name just a few. In addition, when you're fatigued, it is much easier to make a mistake while driving or performing physical activities.

HOW MUCH SLEEP DO WE NEED?

Most doctors agree that adults need between seven and eight hours of sleep a night in order for the body to recover on a cellular level, but it's not only the quantity of sleep that matters; it's also the quality. As we fall asleep, we progress through sleep cycles. Each sleep cycle consists of deep sleep and an REM—rapid eye movement—phase, which is when we dream. As the night progresses, the REM phase becomes longer, which is a critical piece in the biology of sleep. A good night's sleep consists of four to five complete cycles.

There are many things that get in the way of good sleep cycles, including stimulants like caffeine, alcohol, consuming too much light from our screens (phones, tablets, televisions, etc.), or being disturbed by someone else (like a snoring spouse or crying baby). But there are a few measures that Twery suggests you can take to increase your chances of a good night's sleep. He suggests avoiding stimulants such as caffeine and screen time late in the day. Taking part in calming activities at night, such as sipping a cup of herbal tea, taking a bath, or reading, all tend to help us sleep better. Also, use as little light as possible before going to bed in a cool, dark, and quiet room. Healthy exposure to sunlight during the day, consistent exercise, and eating a balanced diet all contribute to the quality of our sleep. Creating a consistent bedtime and wake-up time are also key.

My research inspired me to fine-tune my own routine a little bit. I've made a concerted effort to get off my phone at least thirty minutes before I go to sleep. In addition, I read every night when I crawl into bed, which usually makes me sleepy within minutes! And making my bed physically comfortable with a high-quality mattress, pillows, and bed linens is a wonderful trick, too. When I crawl into bed, I'm in the most relaxing spot in my house.

I'm holding strong on prioritizing my sleep, and I'm willing to bet I feel better for it!

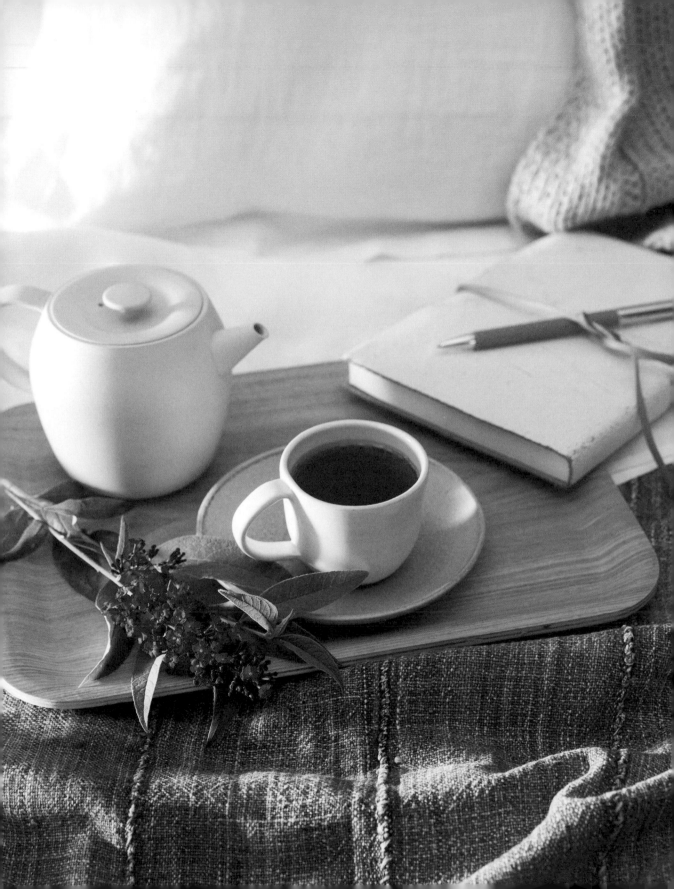

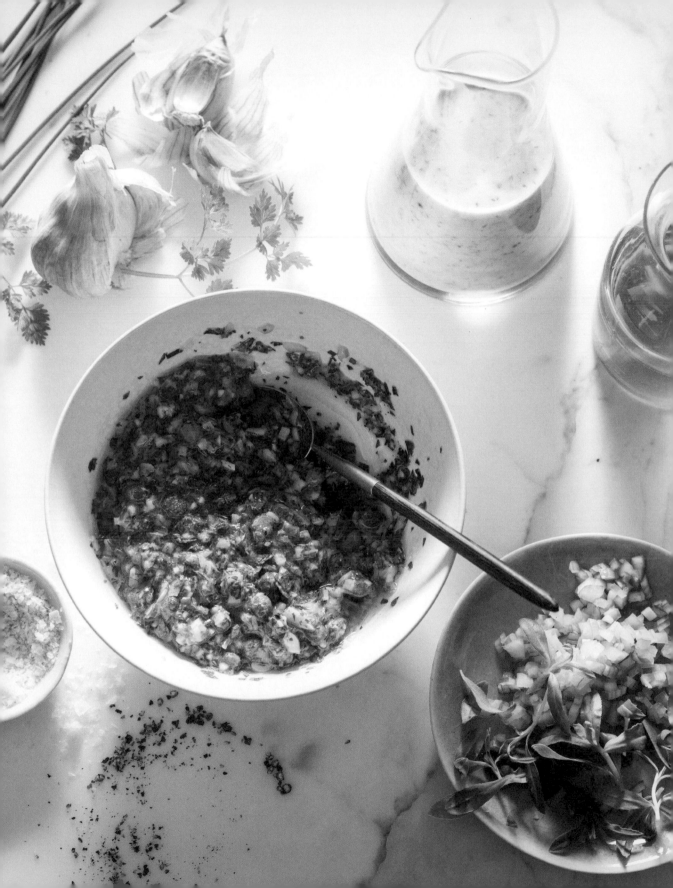

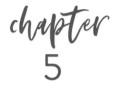

chapter 5

TWELVE STAPLE RECIPES THAT GET ME THROUGH THE WEEK

All cooks have a few recipes they can't live without—the ones they've made so many times they don't even have to think when they make them. For me, these recipes are the ones I keep in my fridge, ready to pull out at any moment to breathe life into the simplest cuts of fish or chicken, or to dollop on scrambled eggs and fried rice. From my green sauces to vinaigrettes to the perfect chicken stock, these recipes are the foundation of my cooking.

SALSA VERDE

I hope with this book, I become known for my green sauces, which my family and friends now affectionately call "Haas Sauces." Chimichurri reigns supreme in my house, but I wanted to do a cutting board version of a green sauce—one where no food processor or blender is required. This one packs a punch with its briny capers, bright citrus, and anti-inflammatory herbs. It's *so easy*. Put it on everything—soups, meat, eggs, grains, you name it.

PREPARATION TIME
10 minutes

MAKES ABOUT
1 cup / 240 ml

2 Tbsp chopped shallot

2 Tbsp capers, rinsed and drained

2 tsp Dijon mustard

2 tsp grated lemon zest,
plus 1 Tbsp fresh lemon juice

1 garlic clove, minced or grated

½ cup [15 g] coarsely chopped
fresh parsley

⅓ cup [15 g] coarsely chopped
fresh mint

⅓ cup [80 ml] extra-virgin olive oil

Kosher salt

Freshly ground black pepper

In a small bowl, stir the shallot, capers, mustard, lemon zest, and garlic with a fork to combine. Add the parsley and mint and stir, then slowly whisk in the oil and lemon juice. Season with salt and pepper. Cover and keep in the refrigerator for up to 1 week.

PRESERVED LEMON GREMOLATA

Typically made with lemon zest, garlic, parsley, and anchovies, this vegan version calls on preserved lemon and salty almonds for depth. The preserved lemon rounds out the clean herbs and bright acid in a way that is downright magical. Spoon this over a baked sweet potato; serve it over grilled shrimp, chicken, or steak; or smother your favorite tacos in it. Oh—it's also delicious over eggs!

PREPARATION TIME
15 minutes

MAKES
1½ cups / 360 g

2 Tbsp white wine vinegar

2 tsp honey

¼ cup [30 g] finely chopped shallot

1 cup [40 g] finely chopped fresh parsley

½ cup [80 g] roasted, salted almonds, finely chopped

2 Tbsp minced preserved lemon, plus 1 tsp preserved lemon liquid

½ cup [120 ml] extra-virgin olive oil

Kosher salt

Freshly ground pepper

In a medium bowl, whisk together the vinegar and honey until the honey dissolves. Stir in the shallot and let sit for 5 minutes. Add the parsley, almonds, lemon and liquid, and oil, and stir to combine. Season with salt and pepper. Serve immediately, or store in an airtight container in the refrigerator for up to 1 week.

HERB BUTTERMILK DRESSING

I love green goddess dressing, but wanted to create something a little lighter. Buttermilk adds the tang and richness I crave, and the mixture of herbs sing together. This dressing is so good on its own, you could simply toss it with butter lettuce or romaine leaves and call it a salad.

PREPARATION TIME
5 minutes

MAKES
3/4 cup / 180 ml

½ cup [120 ml] buttermilk

1 Tbsp fresh lemon juice

½ tsp Dijon mustard

1 garlic clove, minced

2 Tbsp loosely packed fresh parsley leaves

2 Tbsp loosely packed fresh tarragon leaves

2 Tbsp extra-virgin olive oil

2 Tbsp roughly chopped chives

Kosher salt

Freshly ground black pepper

In a food processor, pulse the buttermilk, lemon juice, mustard, and minced garlic to combine. Add the parsley and tarragon and process until smooth and creamy. With the motor running, add the oil in a steady stream until well incorporated. Fold in the chives. Season with salt and pepper. Transfer to an airtight container and store in the refrigerator for up to 1 week.

LEMON VINAIGRETTE

This recipe is a staple in my house. My son Charlie rolls his eyes at me when I ask if he knows how to make it. ("Duh, Mom.") I like a mild olive oil for this so it isn't too assertive. I really want to taste the other ingredients.

PREPARATION TIME
5 minutes

MAKES
1/2 cup / 120 ml

2 Tbsp honey	1/4 cup [60 ml] olive oil
2 Tbsp Dijon mustard	Kosher salt
1/4 cup [60 ml] fresh lemon juice	Freshly ground black pepper

In a medium bowl, whisk the honey and mustard to combine. Whisk in the lemon juice and then the oil. Season with salt and pepper. Serve immediately, or store in an airtight container in the refrigerator for up to 5 days.

LIME VINAIGRETTE

This vinaigrette is wonderful over peaches and arugula with a little goat cheese. It's also a delicious marinade. Add a little chipotle in adobo sauce for heat.

PREPARATION TIME
15 minutes

MAKES
3/4 cup / 180 ml

¼ cup [30 g] minced red onion

1 tsp grated lime zest plus ¼ cup [60 ml] fresh lime juice

1 Tbsp honey

Kosher salt

Freshly ground black pepper

⅓ cup [80 ml] canola oil

In a small bowl, combine the onion, lime zest, and honey. Slowly whisk in the lime juice to dissolve the honey. Season with salt and pepper. Let sit for 10 minutes, so the lime juice softens the red onion a little. Slowly whisk in the oil. Taste and add more salt and pepper as desired. Serve immediately, or store in an airtight container in the refrigerator for up to 5 days.

CURRY AIOLI DRESSING

Calling this "aioli" might be a stretch, as real aioli involves emulsifying egg yolks with olive oil and garlic by whisking as fast as you can. Basically, it's a fancy version of mayonnaise. In this dressing, I wanted to create the consistency of aioli yet pack the anti-inflammatory punch of curry powder. The result is an absolutely delicious twist on aioli—or mayonnaise, if you must.

PREPARATION TIME
5 minutes

MAKES
⅔ cup / 160 ml

2 Tbsp mayonnaise	1 garlic clove, grated
1 Tbsp Dijon mustard	¼ cup [60 ml] olive oil
2 Tbsp fresh lemon juice	Kosher salt
2 tsp curry powder	Freshly ground pepper
2 tsp honey	1 Tbsp water

In a small bowl, whisk the mayonnaise, mustard, lemon juice, curry powder, honey, and garlic to combine. Slowly whisk in the oil. Season with salt and pepper. Whisk in the water to reach a pourable consistency. Taste and add more salt and pepper as desired. Use immediately, or store in an airtight container in the refrigerator for up to 5 days.

CUCUMBER SALAD

with Mint, Red Onion, and Chinese Five Spice

Call this a quick pickle, call it magic . . . I don't care. All I know is that when you put cucumbers and red onions into mirin, they are completely addictive! Eat them on their own, or serve them as a side with any stir-fry, bowl, or grilled meat you make. And cucumbers flush out toxins and keep you hydrated, so think of this recipe whenever you want a little something on the side to perk up your meal!

PREPARATION TIME
15 minutes
(plus 20 minutes to marinate)

SERVES
6

6 Persian cucumbers, unpeeled, scrubbed, and cut into ⅓ in [8 mm] slices on the bias

½ red onion, thinly sliced

2 Tbsp mirin

2 Tbsp rice wine vinegar

1 tsp honey

⅛ tsp Chinese five-spice powder, plus more as needed

Kosher salt

¼ cup [8 g] chopped fresh mint

2 tsp black sesame seeds

Combine the cucumbers, onion, mirin, vinegar, honey, five-spice powder, and a generous pinch of salt in a large bowl. Toss and marinate at room temperature for 20 minutes. Toss in the mint and sesame seeds just before serving, and season with additional salt or five-spice powder as desired. Serve, or transfer to an airtight container and store in the refrigerator for up to 5 days.

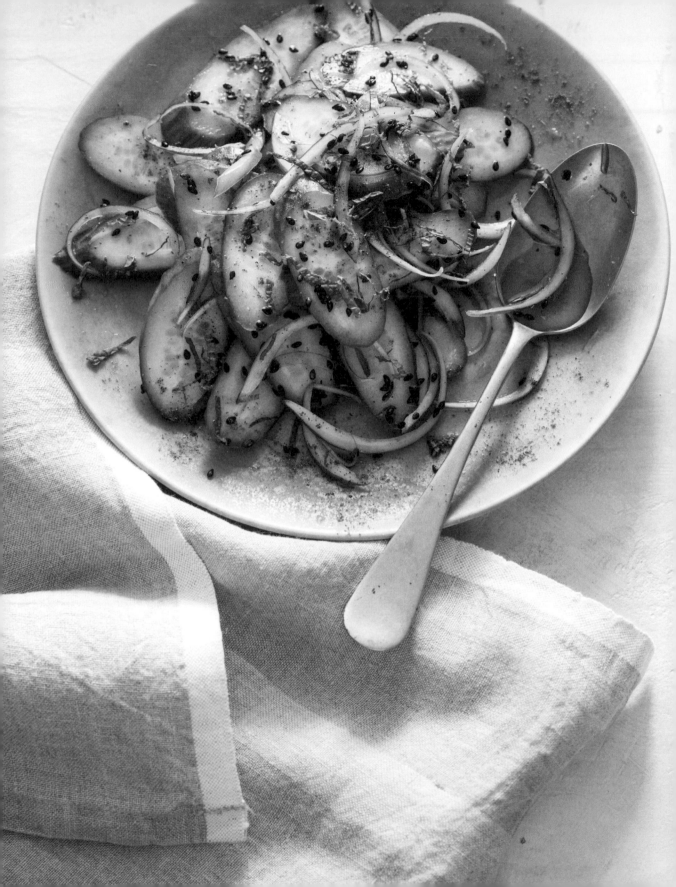

MUSTARD VINAIGRETTE

There is something about the way the French make their vinaigrettes that is special. Simplicity always rules, yet they make sure to add just the right balance of acid and fat. You don't have to include the honey, but I like to add a spoonful to round out the flavors.

PREPARATION TIME
10 minutes

MAKES
¾ cup / 180 ml

2 Tbsp minced shallot

¼ cup [60 ml] fresh lemon juice

2 Tbsp coarse-grain mustard

1 Tbsp honey

½ cup [120 ml] extra-virgin olive oil

Kosher salt

Freshly ground black pepper

In a small bowl, combine the minced shallot with the lemon juice and mustard, and let sit for about 5 minutes. Whisk in the honey. Slowly whisk in the oil until emulsified. Season with salt and pepper. Store in an airtight container in the refrigerator for up to 2 weeks.

TAMARI, GINGER, *and* HONEY MARINADE

(a.k.a. Amanda's Weeknight Marinade)

Looking for salty, sweet, bitter, sour, and umami all in one place? You'll find it with this marinade. This is my go-to marinade for salmon, skirt steak, chicken, and even shrimp. The thing I love is that you only need to marinate fish or shrimp in it for an hour before it's ready to go. You can add chicken or steak to the marinade in the morning if you're serving it for dinner. My trick for avoiding the sodium traps of tamari and soy sauce? I balance a little tamari with a lot of acid from the lime juice and heat from the sriracha.

PREPARATION TIME
5 minutes

MAKES
¾ cup / 180 ml

¼ cup [60 ml] toasted sesame oil	2 Tbsp honey
¼ cup [60 ml] tamari	1 Tbsp grated fresh ginger
1 tsp grated lime zest plus 2 Tbsp fresh lime juice	1 Tbsp sriracha (optional)
	2 garlic cloves, smashed

In a small bowl, whisk together all of the ingredients. Transfer to an airtight container and store in the refrigerator for up to 5 days.

PERFECT CHICKEN STOCK

I'm obsessed with chicken stock. Whether it's the base for my favorite pho at The Slanted Door or used to poach chicken for the best taco I've ever had at Tacubaya in Berkeley, it can transform a dish. And when cooked properly, it's a healing, soothing dish on its own. (I really do think it helps ward off the common cold and other ailments.) The only trick? Simply follow these instructions and be patient. You can't rush perfection, and by golly, it's worth it here. Also, you can cook the chicken whole but you'll need a deeper pot. Simply ask your butcher to cut it into four to six pieces for you and keep the backbone as well. The whole point is to draw the flavor and gelatin out of the bones!

PREPARATION TIME
15 minutes

COOKING TIME
2¼ hours

MAKES ABOUT
12 cups / 2.8 L

One 4 lb [1.8 kg] chicken, cut into 4 pieces, plus the backbone

1 yellow onion, halved

2 garlic cloves, crushed

12 to 14 cups [3 to 3.4 L] cold water

3 tsp kosher salt

Place the chicken pieces, onion, and garlic in a very large stockpot or Dutch oven. Pour in the cold water, adding enough to cover the chicken.

Place over medium heat and slowly bring to a simmer. As soon as it begins to simmer, use a fine-mesh strainer or sieve to skim off any foam that rises to the surface. Cover partially, reduce the heat to low, and simmer for 45 minutes.

Remove the chicken from the pot. Let rest until cool enough to handle, about 10 minutes. Carefully remove the chicken skin and place it back in the pot. Remove all of the meat from the bones, setting the meat aside and returning the bones to the pot. Save the cooked chicken for another use, such as pho (page 137).

Continue to simmer the liquid with the bones and skin for 1 more hour over very low heat, adding more water to ensure the pot is ⅔ full.

Strain the stock through a fine-mesh sieve into a large bowl. It should be fairly bright in color. Stir in 1½ tsp of the salt. Taste, adding the remaining 1½ tsp salt if necessary. Let cool, then transfer to an airtight container and refrigerate for up to 3 days or freeze for up to 1 month.

BASIC QUINOA

When I discovered I was gluten intolerant, I was somewhat forced to love quinoa. I love starchy foods, and was missing things like couscous next to my roast chicken and orzo pasta salad with fresh tomatoes and mozzarella. Quinoa has become the base for some of my best recipes, including the cover photo for my last book! (Who would have thought?!)

This method is the basic preparation of quinoa. I like to make a batch on the weekends, then split it and immediately toss some in vinaigrette to create the base of a salad, then use the rest to toss into stir-fries and my morning breakfast scrambles, or sauté on its own with some olive oil and green onions to create a crispy side dish for whatever I've roasted or grilled that day.

Don't forget to rinse your quinoa before cooking. It will rinse away the saponins, a natural pesticide that many people identify as having a bitter taste.

PREPARATION TIME
5 minutes

COOKING TIME
20 minutes

SERVES
8–10

2 cups [340 g] organic white or red quinoa

4 cups [960 ml] chicken broth, vegetable broth, or water

Pinch of kosher salt

In a fine-mesh strainer, rinse the quinoa well under cold running water and drain.

In a medium saucepan over high heat, bring the chicken broth and salt to a boil. Stir in the quinoa, cover, and turn the heat to medium-low. Simmer until the quinoa is tender and white quinoa tails are visible, about 18 minutes. Transfer to a shallow bowl or baking sheet, and set aside to cool to room temperature. Fluff with a fork, and then serve.

To save for later, cool the quinoa completely before refrigerating. To cool quinoa quickly, spread it out onto a baking sheet. Store in an airtight container in the refrigerator for up to 1 week.

THE PERFECT POACHED EGG

I eat eggs every day of my life for breakfast. I eat them scrambled, fried in olive oil, or my favorite way—poached. Take the time to learn how to poach an egg correctly and it will change your breakfast game forever. And while the water comes to a simmer, you can unload the dishwasher or make yourself a cup of coffee like I do.

PREPARATION TIME
5 minutes

COOKING TIME
3 minutes

SERVES
1

1 Tbsp white vinegar

1 tsp kosher salt

1 fresh egg

Fill a small, shallow saute pan with 1½ in [4 cm] water. Bring to a simmer, then add the vinegar and salt. Lower the temperature so the water is barely bubbling. You should see small bubbles rising to the surface rather than large bubbles popping on top. A rolling boil will cook the eggs too quickly.

Crack the egg into a small bowl or ramekin. (If the yolk breaks, cover the egg with plastic wrap and save for another use.) Gently tip the egg into the water. Cook until the white is barely opaque and the yolk is still runny inside, about 3 minutes.

Using a slotted spoon, gently lift the egg out of the water and place on a paper towel–lined plate. Use the towel to pat off any extra water, then transfer the egg to a dry dish. Serve immediately.

If making poached eggs ahead and not serving them immediately, shock the cooked eggs in a bowl of ice water to stop the cooking. Transfer the ice-water bath and eggs to the refrigerator, and refrigerate for up to 8 hours. To rewarm the eggs, slip them into simmering water and heat for 15 to 30 seconds. Lift them into a strainer to drain, then slide onto a serving plate.

ACKNOWLEDGMENTS

Thank you to . . .

Sarah Billingsley, for picking up the torch with my last book and leading me to this one. I'm forever grateful that you talked me into this idea (but PS, you had me at "hello").

To the incredibly talented team at Chronicle Books, including Laura Lee Mattingly, Sara Schneider, Magnolia Molcan, Steve Kim, and everyone who worked to make this book the best it could be.

The best photo team in the business: Erin Kunkel, your photography inspires me every time I spot it. For me it epitomizes beauty and freedom. George Dolese, your vision for my food is always a better version of my own. If I could pick one person to work with forever, it would be you. Glenn Jenkins, your taste is impeccable. Thank you for creating the beautiful backdrop to make my food sing. The results of your collaborative work are incredible, you three. Thank you for saying yes AGAIN!

Carole Bidnick, for your persistence and belief in my books and in me. Thank you so much.

My testing and development team, whose work can be found throughout these pages. Each one of you brought your own unique style of cooking and passion to this project. Inken Chrisman, Isabelle English, and Emily McFarren, I'm forever grateful for your contributions and can't wait to see where your individual talents take you!

Kate Leahy, all good projects begin with your wisdom and way with words. Our quick meet up was all you needed to lay down a fabulous proposal. Thank you so much for articulating my vision in a way I could not articulate myself. You're magical.

All of my contributors: You made this book the rich, layered guide to good health that I have always wanted to create. Jennifer Aaker, Naomi Bagdonas, Tim Fitzgerald, Denise Henry, Dr. Kelly Hood, Rebecca Katz, Hailey Lott, Stephanie Peters, Dr. Pepper Schwartz, Lindsey Valdez, and Sumner Weldon, you are the reason this book will remain relevant for years to come. Thank you!

Whole Foods Market: Norma Quon, you're my culinary soul sister. Thank you for believing in me more than anyone. I've always believed in the vision of Whole Foods. Every single ingredient I used for this book was found in my local Whole Foods; I am so grateful that you give so many people access to these incredible ingredients.

My Traeger Family: Who knew that I could wake up one morning, look at my Traeger grill, and decide I needed to work with your amazing brand immediately?

Jeremy, it has felt right since the day we spoke. Special thanks to Denny, Brian, Hjalmar, Tina, Amanda, Nichole, Austen, Doug, Shannon, the rest of the incredible Traeger team, and my most trusted and valuable partner in crime, Alisha. I love Traeger's culture and community. Please let me scooter through your office forever!

My Flutie Entertainment Team: Danielle Iturbe, Shab Azma, and Joyce Cavitt—I can't wait for what's to come!

To my mentors and food friends: You all have shaped my career through your guidance, inspiration, and support. Thank you to Tori Ritchie (my original mentor), Keith Belling, Max Borthwick, Stanley Cheng, Katherine Cobbs, Michael Coon, Ayesha Curry, Irene Edwards, Todd English, Jodi Liano, Michael Mina, John Pleasants, and the crew at No Kid Hungry.

Seamus Mullen, you walked into our kitchen when I was at the lowest point with my health. Hours later, after hearing your story, you convinced me that I was completely in control of the outcome. Turns out, you were right! Thank you for sharing your story with the world.

Mr. and Mrs. (Aaker-) Smith: As a couple, you two are my culinary OGs! Thank you for helping me shape my vision oh so many years ago.

Williams-Sonoma: I am so proud of the work we did together and for being lucky enough to share the company's culture with so many new associates. And to the women who now run the world there, thank you for showing all of us what it looks like to persevere in order to achieve your dreams.

Chuck Williams, for providing meaning to my career every day. You were the original dreamer, and the reality of your vision coming to fruition will inspire me for the rest of my life.

And to Me, for remembering that with strength, perseverance, commitment, and belief in myself, all of my dreams are possible—even this one!

REFERENCES

Ingredients for Longevity with Rebecca Katz, MS

Josling, Peter, "Preventing the common cold with a garlic supplement: a double-blind, placebo-controlled survey," *Advances in Natural Therapy* 18, no. 4 (July/August 2001): 189–93, https://www.ncbi.nlm.nih.gov/pubmed/11697022 (accessed November 7, 2018).

Lauretti, Elisabetta, Luigi Iuliano, and Domenico Praticò, "Extra-virgin olive oil ameliorates cognition and neuropathology of the 3xTg mice: role of autophagy," *Annals of Clinical and Translational Neurology* 4, no. 8 (August 2017): 564–74, https://doi.org/10.1002/acn3.431 (accessed November 7, 2018).

Saenghong, Naritsara, Jintanaporn Wattanathorn, Supaporn Muchimapura, Terdthai Tongun, Nawanant Piyavhatkul, Chuleratana Banchonglikitkul, and Tanwarat Kajsongkram, "*Zingiber officinale* Improves Cognitive Function of the Middle-Aged Healthy Women," *Evidence-Based Complementary and Alternative Medicine* 2012 (September 2011): Article ID 383062, https://doi.org/10.1155/2012/383062 (accessed November 7, 2018).

Saenghong, Naritsara, Jintanaporn Wattanathorn, Terdthai Tong-Un, Supaporn Muchimapura, Nawanant Piyavhatkul, Chuleratana Bunchonglikitkul and Tanwarat Kajsongkram, "Ginger Supplementation Enhances Working Memory of the Post-Menopause Women." *American Journal of Applied Sciences* 8, no. 12 (2011): 1241–48, https://pdfs.semanticscholar.org/5459/d16c0cc2247e1a20119adfb2efd91781d8f3.pdf (accessed November 7, 2018).

Time in Nature

"Landmark Report: U.S. Teens Use an Average of Nine Hours of Media Per Day, Tweens Use Six Hours," *Common Sense Media*, November 3, 2015, https://www.commonsensemedia.org/about-us/news/press-releases/landmark-report-us-teens-use-an-average-of-nine-hours-of-media-per-day (accessed November 8, 2018).

Lee, Juyoung, Bum-Jin Park, Yuko Tsunetsugu, Takahide Kagawa, and Yoshifumi Miyazaki, "Restorative effects of viewing real forest landscapes, based on a comparison with urban landscapes," *Scandinavian Journal of Forest Research* 24, no. 3 (June 2009): 227–34, https://doi.org/10.1080/02827580902903341 (accessed on November 8, 2018).

Perez, Sarah, "U.S. Consumers Now Spend 5 Hours per Day on Mobile Devices," *TechCrunch*, 2016, http://tcrn.ch/2mVyWly (accessed November 08, 2018).

Ryan, Richard M., Netta Weinstein, Jessey Bernstein, Kirk Warren Brown, Louis Mistretta, Marylène Gagné, "Vitalizing effects of being outdoors and in nature," *Journal of Environmental Psychology* 30, no. 2 (2010): 159–68, https://doi.org/10.1016/j.jenvp.2009.10.009 (accessed November 7, 2018).

van Praag Gould, Cassandra D., Sarah N. Garfinkel, Oliver Sparasci, Alex Mees, Andrew O. Philippides, Mark Ware, Cristina Ottaviani, and Hugo D. Critchley, "Mind-wandering and alterations to default mode network connectivity when listening to naturalistic versus artificial sounds," *Scientific Reports* 7 (March 2017): Article number 45273, https://doi.org/10.1038/srep45273 (accessed November 7, 2018).

The Medicine of Humor with Dr. Jenifer Aaker and Naomi Bagdanas

Bazzini, Doris G., Elizabeth R. Stack, Penny D. Martincin, and Carmen P. Davis, "The effect of reminiscing about laughter on relationship satisfaction," *Motivation and Emotion* 31, no. 1 (March 2007): 25–34, https://doi.org/10.1007/s11031-006-9045-6 (accessed November 7, 2018).

Beck, Julie, "Funny or Die: How your sense of humor can improve your health, get you pregnant, and even save your life," *The Atlantic Magazine*, June 2014, https://www.theatlantic.com/magazine/archive/2014/06/funny-or-die/361618/#1 (accessed November 8, 2018).

Goh, Joel, Jeffrey Pfeffer, Stefanos Zenios, "The Relationship Between Workplace Stressors and Mortality and Health Costs in the United States," *Management Science* 62, no. 2 (March 2015): 608–28, https://doi.org/10.1287/mnsc.2014.2115 (accessed on November 7, 2018).

Keltner, Dacher, and George Bonanno, "A Study of Laughter and Dissociation: Distinct Correlates of Laughter and Smiling During Bereavement," *Journal of Personality and Social Psychology* 73, no. 4 (April 1997): 687–702, https://www.ncbi.nlm.nih.gov/pubmed/9325589 (accessed November 7, 2018).

Sex and Aging with Pepper Schwartz

Davison, Sonia Louise, Robin Jean Bell, Maria LaChina, Samantha Lee Holden, Susan Ruth Davis, "The Relationship between Self-Reported Sexual Satisfaction and General Well-Being in Women," *The Journal of Sexual Medicine* 6, no. 10 (October 2009): 2690–97, https://doi.org/10.1111/j.1743-6109.2009.01406.x (accessed November 7, 2018).

Fisher, Linda, Gretchen Anderson, Matrika Chapagain, Xenia Montenegro, James Smoot, and Amishi Takalkar, "Sex, Romance, and Relationships," *2009 AARP Survey of Midlife and Older Adults*, May 2010, https://assets.aarp.org /rgcenter/general/srr_09.pdf (accessed November 7, 2018).

Gilbert, Peter, "'I, Robot': has the modern workplace lost its soul?: The context for values based, soul-full leadership," *International Journal of Leadership in Public Services* 7, no. 2 (2011): 77–98, https://doi.org/10.1108/17479881111160078 (accessed November 7, 2018).

Leitzmann, Michael F., Elizabeth A. Platz, Meir J. Stampfer, Walter C. Willett, Edward Giovannucci, "Ejaculation frequency and subsequent risk of prostate cancer," *JAMA* 291, no. 13 (April 2004):1578–86, https://jamanetwork.com/journals /jama/fullarticle/198487 (accessed November 7, 2018).

The Benefits of Acupuncture

"Acupuncture," *NIH Consensus Statement* 15, no. 5 (November 3–5, 1997): 1–34, https://www.ncbi.nlm.nih.gov /pubmed/9809733 (accessed November 8, 2018).

"Acupuncture: Review And Analysis Of Reports On Controlled Clinical Trial," *World Health Organization*, 2003, http://digicollection.org/hss/en/d/Js4926e/ (accessed on November 8, 2018).

Meditation for Self-Love with Hailey Lott

Hölzel, Britta, James Carmody, Mark Vangel, Christina Congleton, Sita Yerramsetti, Tim Gard, and Sara Lazar, "Mindfulness practice leads to increases in regional brain gray matter density," *Psychiatry Research* 191, no. 1 (January 2011): 36–43, https://doi.org/10.1016/j.pscychresns.2010.08.006 (accessed November 7, 2018).

Lazara, Sara, Catherine Kerr, Rachel Wasserman, Jeremy Gray, Douglas Greve, Michael Treadway, Metta McGarvey, Brian Quinn, Jeffery Dusek, Herbert Benson, et al., "Meditation experience is associated with increased cortical thickness," *Neuroreport* 16, no. 17 (November 2005): 1893–97, https://www.ncbi.nlm.nih.gov/pubmed/16272874 (accessed November 7, 2018).

Salzberg, Sharon. *Real Happiness*. New York: Workman Publishing, 2010.

Sleep for Your Health

"The Benefits of Slumber: Why You Need a Good Night's Sleep," *NIH News in Health*, April 2013, https://newsinhealth.nih .gov/2013/04/benefits-slumber (accessed on November 8, 2018).

INDEX

A

Aaker, Jennifer, 107–10
acai berries, 25
    "Haascai" Berry Shakes or Bowls, 25
acupuncture, 128–29
aging
    food and, 52, 54–59
    meditation and, 209–10
    sex and, 122–27
    skin and, 201–2
almond flour
    Almond Flour Banana Bread with Dark Chocolate Chunks, 33
    Chocolate Ganache Tart with Grand Marnier, 181–82
    Gluten-Free Ginger Molasses Cookies, 177
    Summer Berry Pot Pies, 187–88
almond milk
    Coconut-Almond Matcha, 23
    "Haascai" Berry Shakes or Bowls, 25
    Maple-Turmeric Golden Milk, 22
    Strawberry-Basil Smoothies with Almond Milk and Honey, 29
almonds
    Blistered Curry Cauliflower with Mint, Currants, and Toasted Almonds, 93
    Napa Cabbage Salad with Fennel and Roasted Almonds, 73
    Pork and Mango Stir-Fry with Napa Cabbage and Toasted Almonds, 146–47
    Preserved Lemon Gremolata, 221
    Sophia's Toasted Almond Granola with Cardamom and Chocolate Chunks, 27
    Strawberry-Arugula Salad with Toasted Almonds and Mint, 72
    Thai Rice Noodles with Peppers and Asparagus, 85–87
Amanda's California Cocktail, 195
animal protein, 131–32
antioxidants, 204–5, 206
Apples, Warm Spinach Salad with Beets, Bacon Vinaigrette, and, 79
apricots
    Late Summer Salad with Heirloom Tomatoes, Stone Fruit, Goat Cheese, and Pistachios, 81
    Stone Fruit and Berry Crisp, 178
aromatherapy massage, 64
arugula
    Fall Quinoa Salad with Butternut Squash, Toasted Pepitas, and Raisins, 101
    Strawberry-Arugula Salad with Toasted Almonds and Mint, 72
Asian pears
    Butter Lettuce Salad with Asian Pears, Pistachios, and Pomegranate Seeds, 75
    Meyer Lemon and Asian Pear Juice with Mint, 26
Asparagus, Thai Rice Noodles with Peppers and, 85–87
avocados, 54–55
    Ceviche with Grilled Pineapple, Tomatillos, and Jalapeño, 167
    Modern Salade Niçoise with Poached Tuna and Curry Aioli Dressing, 77–78
    "Stir-Fried" Quinoa and Greens with Poached Eggs, Avocado, and Salsa Verde, 38–39

B

Bacon Vinaigrette, Warm Spinach Salad with Beets, Apples, and, 79
Bagdonas, Naomi, 107–10
Banana Bread, Almond Flour, with Dark Chocolate Chunks, 33
beans
    Green Bean and Snap Pea Salad with Mustard Vinaigrette, 83–84

    Lentil Minestrone with Chard, White Beans, and (Sometimes) Sausage, 90–91
    Merritt's Sexy Cannellini Beans (a.k.a. Almost-Vegetarian Cassoulet), 97–98
    Modern Salade Niçoise with Poached Tuna and Curry Aioli Dressing, 77–78
    Sweet Potato–Turkey Chili with Cilantro Oil and Pepitas, 149–50
beef
    grass-fed, 131–32, 155
    Grilled Rib Eyes with Hasselback Sweet Potatoes and Preserved Lemon Gremolata, 155–56
    Steak Tacos with Cabbage Slaw, Mango Salsa, and Chipotle Mayonnaise, 157–59
Beets, Warm Spinach Salad with Apples, Bacon Vinaigrette, and, 79
Belcampo Meats, 132, 155
bell peppers
    Crustless Mini-Quiches with Roasted Red Pepper, Basil, and Goat Cheese, 35
    Thai Rice Noodles with Peppers and Asparagus, 85–87
berries. See also individual berries
    Stone Fruit and Berry Crisp, 178
    Summer Berry Pot Pies, 187–88
Blodgett, Leslie, 109
blueberries
    Buckwheat Crêpes with Berry Compote and Maple-Whipped Goat Cheese, 36–37
    Summer Berry Pot Pies, 187–88
Bok Choy, Coconut Ginger Sea Bass in Parchment with King Trumpet Mushrooms and, 160–62
Borthwick, Max, 172
Bread, Almond Flour Banana, with Dark Chocolate Chunks, 33
breathwork, 42–43
Brussels Sprouts, Shaved, with Root Vegetables and Citrus–Goat Cheese Vinaigrette, 99
Buckwheat Crêpes with Berry Compote and Maple-Whipped Goat Cheese, 36–37
Burger, Thai Chicken, with Pickled Papaya Slaw, 144–45
burpees, 112
Butcher Box, 132

C

cabbage
    Cabbage Slaw, 157–59
    Napa Cabbage Salad with Fennel and Roasted Almonds, 73
    Pork and Mango Stir-Fry with Napa Cabbage and Toasted Almonds, 146–47
cashew milk
    Chai-Spiced Cashew Milk, 24
    Maple-Turmeric Golden Milk, 22
Cat/Cow, 45–46
cauliflower
    Blistered Curry Cauliflower with Mint, Currants, and Toasted Almonds, 93
    Cauliflower-Kale Soup with Toasted Pine Nuts, 95–96
    Roasted Moroccan Chicken with Cauliflower "Couscous," 139–41
cayenne, 57
Ceviche with Grilled Pineapple, Tomatillos, and Jalapeño, 167
Chai-Spiced Cashew Milk, 24
chard
    Lentil Minestrone with Chard, White Beans, and (Sometimes) Sausage, 90–91
    "Stir-Fried" Quinoa and Greens with Poached Eggs, Avocado, and Salsa Verde, 38–39

cheese
    Buckwheat Crêpes with Berry Compote and Maple-Whipped Goat Cheese, 36–37
    Crustless Mini-Quiches with Roasted Red Pepper, Basil, and Goat Cheese, 35
    Late Summer Salad with Heirloom Tomatoes, Stone Fruit, Goat Cheese, and Pistachios, 81
    Shaved Brussels Sprouts with Root Vegetables and Citrus-Goat Cheese Vinaigrette, 99
    Warm Spinach Salad with Beets, Apples, and Bacon Vinaigrette, 79
    Zucchini "Spaghetti" with Corn and Cherry Tomatoes, 103
Chermoula, 140, 141
cherries
    Chocolate Ganache Tart with Grand Marnier, 181–82
    Greek Frozen Yogurt with Luxardo Cherries and Dark Chocolate Chunks, 179
    Sophia's Toasted Almond Granola with Cardamom and Chocolate Chunks, 27
    Tequila Old-Fashioneds with Luxardo Cherries, 191
    Wild Rice Salad with Butternut Squash, Cherries, and Mint, 105
chicken
    Chicken in Lettuce Cups with Crispy Pine Nuts and Lime, 133–34
    Chicken Pho with Daikon "Noodles," 137–38
    Perfect Chicken Stock, 230
    Roasted Moroccan Chicken with Cauliflower "Couscous," 139–41
    Sticky Orange Chicken with Caramelized Onions and Fennel, 142
    Thai Chicken Burger with Pickled Papaya Slaw, 144–45
Child's Pose, 46, 48
Chili, Sweet Potato-Turkey, with Cilantro Oil and Pepitas, 149–50
Chipotle Mayonnaise, 159
chocolate
    Almond Flour Banana Bread with Dark Chocolate Chunks, 33
    Chocolate Ganache Tart with Grand Marnier, 181–82
    Greek Frozen Yogurt with Luxardo Cherries and Dark Chocolate Chunks, 179
    Sophia's Toasted Almond Granola with Cardamom and Chocolate Chunks, 27
Chow, 151
Chrisman, Inken, 190
Cilantro Oil, 149–50
cinnamon, 57
citrus, 58–59. See also individual fruits
Cobra Pose, 48
cocktails
    Amanda's California Cocktail, 195
    Herb Garden Gin and Tonic, 192
    Sauvignon Blanc Sangria, 194
    Tequila Old-Fashioneds with Luxardo Cherries, 191
coconut
    Coconut-Almond Matcha, 23
    Coconut Ginger Sea Bass in Parchment with King Trumpet Mushrooms and Bok Choy, 160–62
    Coconut Thai Prawns with Turmeric and Ginger, 172–73
    Matcha Panna Cotta, 183–85
cold therapy. See cyrotherapy
Collinge, William, 200
Cookies, Gluten-Free Ginger Molasses, 177
corn
    Pan-Seared Scallops with Citrusy Corn Succotash, 168
    Zucchini "Spaghetti" with Corn and Cherry Tomatoes, 103
Corpse Pose, 51
cranberries
    Cranberry Sauce, 151–52
    Sophia's Toasted Almond Granola with Cardamom and Chocolate Chunks, 27
Crêpes, Buckwheat, with Berry Compote and Maple-Whipped Goat Cheese, 36–37
Crisp, Stone Fruit and Berry, 178
cucumbers
    Cucumber Salad with Mint, Red Onion, and Chinese Five Spice, 226
    Pickled Cucumber, 163–65
cumin, 57
currants
    Blistered Curry Cauliflower with Mint, Currants, and Toasted Almonds, 93
    Currant Brown Butter Sauce, 170–71

Curry Aioli Dressing, 77–78, 225
cyrotherapy, 120–21

D
Daikon "Noodles," Chicken Pho with, 137–38
deep tissue massage, 64
desserts
    Chocolate Ganache Tart with Grand Marnier, 181–82
    Gluten-Free Ginger Molasses Cookies, 177
    Greek Frozen Yogurt with Luxardo Cherries and Dark Chocolate Chunks, 179
    Matcha Panna Cotta, 183–85
    Orange-Tarragon Granita, 190
    Stone Fruit and Berry Crisp, 178
    Summer Berry Pot Pies, 187–88
dips (exercise), 117
Dirty Dozen, 15
dopamine, 124
Downward-Facing Dog, 47
drinks. See also cocktails
    Chai-Spiced Cashew Milk, 24
    Coconut-Almond Matcha, 23
    "Haascai" Berry Shakes or Bowls, 25
    Maple-Turmeric Golden Milk, 22
    Meyer Lemon and Asian Pear Juice with Mint, 26
    Strawberry-Basil Smoothies with Almond Milk and Honey, 29

E
eggs
    Crustless Mini-Quiches with Roasted Red Pepper, Basil, and Goat Cheese, 35
    Modern Salade Niçoise with Poached Tuna and Curry Aioli Dressing, 77–78
    The Perfect Poached Egg, 232
    Sheet-Pan Smoky Sweet Potato Hash with Oven-Roasted Eggs, 31
    "Stir-Fried" Quinoa and Greens with Poached Eggs, Avocado, and Salsa Verde, 38–39
English, Belle, 160, 177
exercise
    group, 197–200
    motivation for, 200
    in nature, 62
    strength training, 111–19

F
Fall Quinoa Salad with Butternut Squash, Toasted Pepitas, and Raisins, 101
fennel
    Napa Cabbage Salad with Fennel and Roasted Almonds, 73
    Sticky Orange Chicken with Caramelized Onions and Fennel, 142
Fernald, Anya, 132
fish
    Ceviche with Grilled Pineapple, Tomatillos, and Jalapeño, 167
    Coconut Ginger Sea Bass in Parchment with King Trumpet Mushrooms and Bok Choy, 160–62
    Modern Salade Niçoise with Poached Tuna and Curry Aioli Dressing, 77–78
    Tuna Poke with Miso Mayonnaise and Pickled Cucumber, 163–65
    Whole-Roasted Fish with Currant Brown Butter Sauce, 170–71
Fitzgerald, Tim, 120–21
Flat Back, 49
food philosophy, 14–15
Forward Fold, 49
free radicals, 55
French Laundry, 179
friendship, 123–24

G
Garden Day Network, 131
garlic, 58
Gerber, Rande, 191
Gin and Tonic, Herb Garden, 192
ginger, 57
    Gluten-Free Ginger Molasses Cookies, 177
Goh, Joel, 108

Grand Marnier
    Chocolate Ganache Tart with Grand Marnier, 181–82
    Sauvignon Blanc Sangria, 194
Granita, Orange-Tarragon, 190
Granola, Sophia's Toasted Almond, with Cardamom and Chocolate
    Chunks, 27
Greek Frozen Yogurt with Luxardo Cherries and Dark Chocolate
    Chunks, 179
greens, 58. *See also individual greens*
Gremolata, Preserved Lemon, 221
group exercise, 197–200

H

"Haascai" Berry Shakes or Bowls, 25
halibut
    Ceviche with Grilled Pineapple, Tomatillos, and Jalapeño, 167
Henry, Denise, 111–19
herbs, 56. *See also individual herbs*
    Herb Buttermilk Dressing, 222
    Herb Garden Gin and Tonic, 192
Hood, Kelly, 201–2, 204–6
hot stone massage, 64
humor, 107–10

I

inflammation, 14–15, 57–58
ingredients, 16–17

J

jump lunges, 116

K

Kale Soup, Cauliflower-, with Toasted Pine Nuts, 95–96
Katz, Rebecca, 52, 54–59, 71
King, Gayle, 101
Kvochak, Sophia, 27

L

laughter, 107–10
Lawson, Nigella, 142
Lazar, Sara, 209
lemons
    Lemon Vinaigrette, 223
    Meyer Lemon and Asian Pear Juice with Mint, 26
    Preserved Lemon Gremolata, 221
Lentil Minestrone with Chard, White Beans, and (Sometimes) Sausage,
    90–91
letting go, 211
lettuce
    Butter Lettuce Salad with Asian Pears, Pistachios, and Pomegranate
        Seeds, 75
    Chicken in Lettuce Cups with Crispy Pine Nuts and Lime, 133–34
    Modern Salade Niçoise with Poached Tuna and Curry Aioli Dressing,
        77–78
limes
    Chicken in Lettuce Cups with Crispy Pine Nuts and Lime, 133–34
    Lime Vinaigrette, 224
    Pan-Seared Scallops with Citrusy Corn Succotash, 168
Lott, Hailey, 207, 209–14
Low Push-Up, 48

M

mangoes
    "Haascai" Berry Shakes or Bowls, 25
    Mango Salsa, 159
    Pork and Mango Stir-Fry with Napa Cabbage and Toasted Almonds,
        146–47
Maple-Turmeric Golden Milk, 22
Marinade, Tamari, Ginger, and Honey (a.k.a. Amanda's Weeknight
    Marinade), 229
massage therapy, 63–64, 66–67
matcha, 23
    Coconut-Almond Matcha, 23
    Matcha Panna Cotta, 183–85
mayonnaise
    Chipotle Mayonnaise, 159
    Miso Mayonnaise, 163–65

meditation, 207, 209–14
menopause, 126–27
mental energy, restoring, 62
mental health, improving, 62
Merritt's Sexy Cannellini Beans (a.k.a. Almost-Vegetarian Cassoulet),
    97–98
Meyer Lemon and Asian Pear Juice with Mint, 26
Minestrone, Lentil, with Chard, White Beans, and (Sometimes) Sausage,
    90–91
mint, 56
    Blistered Curry Cauliflower with Mint, Currants, and Toasted
        Almonds, 93
    Cucumber Salad with Mint, Red Onion, and Chinese Five Spice, 226
    Meyer Lemon and Asian Pear Juice with Mint, 26
    Salsa Verde, 220
    Strawberry-Arugula Salad with Toasted Almonds and Mint, 72
    Wild Rice Salad with Butternut Squash, Cherries, and Mint, 105
Miso Mayonnaise, 163–65
Mitler, Merrill, 215
mountain climbers, 119
Mountain Pose, 49
Mullen, Seamus, 11–12, 88
mushrooms
    Chicken in Lettuce Cups with Crispy Pine Nuts and Lime, 133–34
    Coconut Ginger Sea Bass in Parchment with King Trumpet
        Mushrooms and Bok Choy, 160–62
Mustard Vinaigrette, 83–84, 228

N

National Alliance on Mental Illness, 69
National Institute of Mental Health, 69
nature, time in, 61–62
nectarines
    Late Summer Salad with Heirloom Tomatoes, Stone Fruit, Goat
        Cheese, and Pistachios, 81
Stone Fruit and Berry Crisp, 178
Nihill, David, 109
noodles
    Coconut Thai Prawns with Turmeric and Ginger, 172–73
    Thai Rice Noodles with Peppers and Asparagus, 85–87

O

oats
    Sophia's Toasted Almond Granola with Cardamom and Chocolate
        Chunks, 27
    Stone Fruit and Berry Crisp, 178
oil
    Cilantro Oil, 149–50
    olive, 55
Old-Fashioneds, Tequila, with Luxardo Cherries, 191
onions
    Cucumber Salad with Mint, Red Onion, and Chinese Five Spice, 226
    Sticky Orange Chicken with Caramelized Onions and Fennel, 142
Opposite Arm, Opposite Leg, 47
oranges
    Citrus–Goat Cheese Vinaigrette, 99
    Orange-Tarragon Granita, 190
    Sticky Orange Chicken with Caramelized Onions and Fennel, 142
organic food, 15
Ottolenghi, Yotam, 83
oxytocin, 108, 124

P

Panna Cotta, Matcha, 183–85
Papaya Slaw, Pickled, Thai Chicken Burger with, 144–45
parsley, 56
    Preserved Lemon Gremolata, 221
    Salsa Verde, 220
parsnips
    Shaved Brussels Sprouts with Root Vegetables and Citrus–Goat
        Cheese Vinaigrette, 99
peaches
    Late Summer Salad with Heirloom Tomatoes, Stone Fruit, Goat
        Cheese, and Pistachios, 81
    Stone Fruit and Berry Crisp, 178
Pea Salad, Snap, Green Bean and, with Mustard Vinaigrette, 83–84

pepitas
  Fall Quinoa Salad with Butternut Squash, Toasted Pepitas, and Raisins, 101
  Sophia's Toasted Almond Granola with Cardamom and Chocolate Chunks, 27
  Sweet Potato–Turkey Chili with Cilantro Oil and Pepitas, 149–50
Peters, Stephanie, 197–200
Pfeffer, Jeff, 108
Phan, Charles, 137
Pho, Chicken, with Daikon "Noodles," 137–38
Pineapple, Grilled, Ceviche with Tomatillos, Jalapeño, and, 167
pine nuts
  Cauliflower-Kale Soup with Toasted Pine Nuts, 95–96
  Chicken in Lettuce Cups with Crispy Pine Nuts and Lime, 133–34
  Currant Brown Butter Sauce, 170–71
pistachios
  Butter Lettuce Salad with Asian Pears, Pistachios, and Pomegranate Seeds, 75
  Chocolate Ganache Tart with Grand Marnier, 181–82
  Late Summer Salad with Heirloom Tomatoes, Stone Fruit, Goat Cheese, and Pistachios, 81
  Wild Rice Salad with Butternut Squash, Cherries, and Mint, 105
Plank Pose, 48
planks, 113–14
plums
  Late Summer Salad with Heirloom Tomatoes, Stone Fruit, Goat Cheese, and Pistachios, 81
  Stone Fruit and Berry Crisp, 178
pomegranates
  Butter Lettuce Salad with Asian Pears, Pistachios, and Pomegranate Seeds, 75
  Shaved Brussels Sprouts with Root Vegetables and Citrus–Goat Cheese Vinaigrette, 99
pork
  Pork and Mango Stir-Fry with Napa Cabbage and Toasted Almonds, 146–47
  Pork Chops with Mashed Sweet Potatoes and Cranberry Sauce, 151–53
Pot Pies, Summer Berry, 187–88
pranayama, 42–43
Prawns, Coconut Thai, with Turmeric and Ginger, 172–73
push-ups, 114–15

Q
Quiches, Crustless Mini-, with Roasted Red Pepper, Basil, and Goat Cheese, 35
quinoa
  Basic Quinoa, 231
  Fall Quinoa Salad with Butternut Squash, Toasted Pepitas, and Raisins, 101
  "Stir-Fried" Quinoa and Greens with Poached Eggs, Avocado, and Salsa Verde, 38–39
  Strawberry-Arugula Salad with Toasted Almonds and Mint, 72

R
radicchio
  Modern Salade Niçoise with Poached Tuna and Curry Aioli Dressing, 77–78
raisins
  Currant Brown Butter Sauce, 170–71
  Fall Quinoa Salad with Butternut Squash, Toasted Pepitas, and Raisins, 101
raspberries
  Matcha Panna Cotta, 183–85
  Sauvignon Blanc Sangria, 194
  Stone Fruit and Berry Crisp, 178
  Summer Berry Pot Pies, 187–88
Reclined Bound Angle Pose, 44
reflexology, 67
relationships, 123–24
retinoids, 204, 206
reverse crunches, 118

S
salad dressings. See also vinaigrettes
  Curry Aioli Dressing, 77–78, 225
  Herb Buttermilk Dressing, 222

salads
  Butter Lettuce Salad with Asian Pears, Pistachios, and Pomegranate Seeds, 75
  Cabbage Slaw, 157–59
  Cucumber Salad with Mint, Red Onion, and Chinese Five Spice, 226
  Fall Quinoa Salad with Butternut Squash, Toasted Pepitas, and Raisins, 101
  Green Bean and Snap Pea Salad with Mustard Vinaigrette, 83–84
  Late Summer Salad with Heirloom Tomatoes, Stone Fruit, Goat Cheese, and Pistachios, 81
  Modern Salade Niçoise with Poached Tuna and Curry Aioli Dressing, 77–78
  Napa Cabbage Salad with Fennel and Roasted Almonds, 73
  Pickled Papaya Slaw, 144–45
  Shaved Brussels Sprouts with Root Vegetables and Citrus–Goat Cheese Vinaigrette, 99
  Strawberry-Arugula Salad with Toasted Almonds and Mint, 72
  Warm Spinach Salad with Beets, Apples, and Bacon Vinaigrette, 79
  Wild Rice Salad with Butternut Squash, Cherries, and Mint, 105
salsas. See sauces and salsas
Salzberg, Sharon, 209
Sangria, Sauvignon Blanc, 194
sauces and salsas
  Cranberry Sauce, 151–52
  Currant Brown Butter Sauce, 170–71
  Mango Salsa, 159
  Salsa Verde, 220
Sausage, Lentil Minestrone with Chard, White Beans, and (Sometimes), 90–91
Sauvignon Blanc Sangria, 194
Scallops, Pan-Seared, with Citrusy Corn Succotash, 168
Schwartz, Pepper, 12, 13, 122–27
Sea Bass, Coconut Ginger, in Parchment with King Trumpet Mushrooms and Bok Choy, 160–62
Seamus's Butternut Squash Soup with Garlicky Panko Crumbs, 88–89
self-love, meditation for, 207, 209–14
sex, 122–27
Shakes, "Haascai" Berry, 25
Shavasana, 51
shiatsu massage, 66
skin care, 201–2, 204–6
The Slanted Door, 137, 230
sleep, 215–16
Smoothies, Strawberry-Basil, with Almond Milk and Honey, 29
Snake River Farms, 132
Sophia's Toasted Almond Granola with Cardamom and Chocolate Chunks, 27
SoulCycle, 197, 198, 200
soups
  Cauliflower-Kale Soup with Toasted Pine Nuts, 95–96
  Chicken Pho with Daikon "Noodles," 137–38
  Lentil Minestrone with Chard, White Beans, and (Sometimes) Sausage, 90–91
  Seamus's Butternut Squash Soup with Garlicky Panko Crumbs, 88–89
Souvla, 179
spices, 57–58
Spinach Salad, Warm, with Beets, Apples, and Bacon Vinaigrette, 79
sports medicine massage, 67
squash
  Fall Quinoa Salad with Butternut Squash, Toasted Pepitas, and Raisins, 101
  Seamus's Butternut Squash Soup with Garlicky Panko Crumbs, 88–89
  Wild Rice Salad with Butternut Squash, Cherries, and Mint, 105
  Zucchini "Spaghetti" with Corn and Cherry Tomatoes, 103
squats, 113
step-ups, 115
St-Germain liqueur
  Amanda's California Cocktail, 195
Stock, Perfect Chicken, 230
strawberries
  Buckwheat Crêpes with Berry Compote and Maple-Whipped Goat Cheese, 36–37
  "Haascai" Berry Shakes or Bowls, 25
  Strawberry-Arugula Salad with Toasted Almonds and Mint, 72

Strawberry-Basil Smoothies with Almond Milk and Honey, 29
Summer Berry Pot Pies, 187–88
strength training, 111–19
stress, reducing, 62
sugar, 175, 205
Summer Berry Pot Pies, 187–88
Sun Breaths, 49–50
sun exposure, 201, 202, 204
Supine Twist, 45
Swedish massage, 63
sweet potatoes
    Grilled Rib Eyes with Hasselback Sweet Potatoes and Preserved
        Lemon Gremolata, 155–56
    Pork Chops with Mashed Sweet Potatoes and Cranberry Sauce,
        151–53
    Shaved Brussels Sprouts with Root Vegetables and Citrus–Goat
        Cheese Vinaigrette, 99
    Sheet-Pan Smoky Sweet Potato Hash with Oven-Roasted Eggs, 31
    Sweet Potato–Turkey Chili with Cilantro Oil and Pepitas, 149–50

T
Tacos, Steak, with Cabbage Slaw, Mango Salsa, and Chipotle
    Mayonnaise, 157–59
Tacubaya, 230
Tamari, Ginger, and Honey Marinade (a.k.a. Amanda's Weeknight
    Marinade), 229
Tart, Chocolate Ganache, with Grand Marnier, 181–82
Tequila Old-Fashioneds with Luxardo Cherries, 191
Thai Chicken Burger with Pickled Papaya Slaw, 144–45
Thai massage, 66
Thai Rice Noodles with Peppers and Asparagus, 85–87
therapy, 68–69
Thornton, Sally, 109
Tomatillos, Ceviche with Grilled Pineapple, Jalapeño, and, 167
tomatoes
    Late Summer Salad with Heirloom Tomatoes, Stone Fruit, Goat
        Cheese, and Pistachios, 81
    Lentil Minestrone with Chard, White Beans, and (Sometimes)
        Sausage, 90–91
    Pan-Seared Scallops with Citrusy Corn Succotash, 168
    Sweet Potato–Turkey Chili with Cilantro Oil and Pepitas, 149–50
    Zucchini "Spaghetti" with Corn and Cherry Tomatoes, 103
tools, 17–19
tortillas
    Fried Tortilla Strips, 150
    Steak Tacos with Cabbage Slaw, Mango Salsa, and Chipotle
        Mayonnaise, 157–59
tuna
    Modern Salade Niçoise with Poached Tuna and Curry Aioli Dressing,
        77–78
    Tuna Poke with Miso Mayonnaise and Pickled Cucumber, 163–65
Turkey Chili, Sweet Potato–, with Cilantro Oil and Pepitas, 149–50
turmeric, 57–58
Twery, Michael, 215, 216

V
Valdez, Lindsey, 41–51
vegetables, 54. *See also individual vegetables*
vinaigrettes
    Citrus–Goat Cheese Vinaigrette, 99
    Lemon Vinaigrette, 223
    Lime Vinaigrette, 224
    Mustard Vinaigrette, 83–84, 228
Vinyasa, 48
vitamins
    A, 55, 205
    C, 205
    D, 55, 202
    E, 55, 205
    K, 55
vodka
    Amanda's California Cocktail, 195

W
Watts, Merritt, 97
Weldon, Sumner, 197–200
Wild Rice Salad with Butternut Squash, Cherries, and Mint, 105

wine
    Sauvignon Blanc Sangria, 194

Y
Yamaguchi, Toshima, 120
yoga
    benefits of, 41–42
    pranayama, 42–43
    sequence for daily practice, 43–51
Yogurt, Greek Frozen, with Luxardo Cherries and Dark Chocolate
    Chunks, 179

Z
Zenios, Stefanos, 108
Zucchini "Spaghetti" with Corn and Cherry Tomatoes, 103